Mekong Me

Mekong Medicine

*A U.S. Doctor's Year Treating
Vietnam's Forgotten Victims*

RICHARD W. CARLSON, M.D.

McFarland & Company, Inc., Publishers
Jefferson, North Carolina

LIBRARY OF CONGRESS CATALOGUING-IN-PUBLICATION DATA

Names: Carlson, Richard W., author.
Title: Mekong medicine : a U.S. doctor's year treating Vietnam's forgotten victims /
Richard W. Carlson, M.D..
Description: Jefferson, North Carolina : McFarland & Company, Inc., Publishers, 2022 |
Includes bibliographical references and index.
Identifiers: LCCN 2022026870 | ISBN 9781476687896 (paperback : acid free paper) ∞
ISBN 9781476646022 (ebook)
Subjects: LCSH: Carlson, Richard W. | Vietnam War, 1961-1975—Medical care. |
Vietnam War, 1961-1975—Personal narratives, American. | Physicians—
United States—Biography. | Humanitarian assistance—Vietnam—Bạc Liêu (Province)—
History—20th century. | United States. Army—Medical personnel—Biography. |
Military Provincial Health Assistance Program (U.S.) | Bạc Liêu (Vietnam : Province)—
History—20th century. | BISAC: HISTORY / Wars & Conflicts / Vietnam War |
MEDICAL / History
Classification: LCC DS559.44 .C37 2022 | DDC 959.704/37092 [B]—dc23/eng/20220607
LC record available at https://lccn.loc.gov/2022026870

BRITISH LIBRARY CATALOGUING DATA ARE AVAILABLE

ISBN (print) 978-1-4766-8789-6
ISBN (ebook) 978-1-4766-4602-2

Front cover: *inset* Author, ready for the day;
background photograph of Mekong river (Shutterstock/high fliers)

Printed in the United States of America

*McFarland & Company, Inc., Publishers
Box 611, Jefferson, North Carolina 28640
www.mcfarlandpub.com*

For Barbara with Love

Acknowledgments

Many people have helped with this project since Barbara suggested I review my Vietnam journal.

Laura Carlson, PhD, and Michael Portt: Love and invaluable assistance; many suggestions, aid on multiple topics; incredible expertise with files and programs.

April Aguiñaga, Maricopa-Valleywise Medical Library: Unending support; a detective for obscure references and citations.

Rebecca Birr, Maricopa-Valleywise Medical Library: Citations, encouragement; guided me to Valerie Danner.

Arizona Military Museum: Access to a 105 mm howitzer.

Judy Hodgkins: Forever helpful; strained eyes to retype faded images.

Katharine Villard, PhD: Love and early tips from an editor.

Amber Dushman, AMA Research Department: VPVN program; a copy of my *Bac Si My* film.

University of Southern California Alumni Staff: Found Dr. Francis Reynard; key historical data on USC and LA County Hospital.

Drexel-Hahnemann University Alumni Association: Help documenting Dr. Charles Gueriera.

Francis Reynard, MD: Invaluable details of Steve and the Vinhs.

Robert Iverson, MD: Motivation, suggestions, and a shared VN experience.

Robert Brittis, MD, Juliana Brittis: A treasure of details, assistance, and photos; the key to Dr. Jim Jones.

Bonnie and Charlie Pratt: Love and everlasting faith.

Marilyn Haupt, MD: Reviewed early drafts, many helpful suggestions.

Tracy Cooper, Jackie Gill, and Deb Hanauer: Support during a difficult time.

Joseph Neal, MD: Source of new facts, especially of Dr. Jim Jones; encouragement

The Pezzi family, especially Christopher Pezzi, MD: Graciously shared their father's inspiring life and his final thoughts of VN.

Valerie Danner: My heroine; volunteered her skills tirelessly, meaningful advice, great editorial suggestions. Many thanks.

Table of Contents

Preface

This book documents a year of my life as a U.S. Army physician, working in a provincial hospital in Vietnam's Mekong Delta caring for civilians as war swirled around me. The text is a firsthand account of my experiences from November 1966 to October 1967. While in Vietnam the portable typewriter that I had brought from Los Angeles became my friend. Each night I religiously recorded the day's events and conversations. The narrative and conversations provided within this book are contemporaneous as I recorded them. I have added subsequent comments, explanations, and descriptions to provide context and to clarify medical, military, or historical topics.

An amazing cast of characters populated my Vietnam odyssey, making the journey more interesting. The people described herein are real. Sensitive facts and some personal information have been edited, but the exploits of these remarkable, often inspiring individuals are true. I have been able to trace the subsequent lives of some with the help of information in the public record, organizations, or families. My search for others has been unsuccessful. The names of a few individuals have not been exposed to protect their identity.

My journal recounts our battles with trauma and disease as we attempted to achieve some normalcy during the war's maelstrom. The tedium and the terrifying coexisted—aligning memorable with the inane. It was an uneven journey, but one of discovery. We experienced personal triumphs as well as tragedies and monumental failures.

The Vietnam War dramatically altered or extinguished millions of lives. The story I tell is one of helping people despite formidable odds.

1

November 1966

Prelude to Bac Lieu, Finding My Footing

San Francisco was cold, damp, and surrounded by a fog that obscured the city's famous skyline. Many soldiers arrived in Vietnam via military aircraft; I was among the lucky to fly a commercial airliner, complete with flight attendants.

It was late 1966. Life in America was juxtaposed with the silly—*Batman* aired on TV and the miniskirt and bikini were wildly popular—and the prophetic: In March, the first major anti–Vietnam War protests erupted, related to the news U.S. troop strength would sharply increase. In June, America initiated bombing of Hanoi and U.S. involvement in Vietnam that had seen the leadership of three presidents entered its second decade. I was about to join the effort.

My brother and his wife, Kathie, accompanied me to transport my dunnage to nearby Travis Air Force Base. The military terminal was like any other commercial airport, except for large numbers of uniformed people and the lack of the usual noise of a busy venue. The atmosphere was tense and artificial. People stood in small groups, checking their watches every few minutes against a large wall clock displaying times around the world. Many soldiers sat on benches, trying to look unconcerned; others stared blankly. Collections of three or four men chatted as they leaned against pillars. Occasionally, an outburst of laughter punctuated the quiet, startling the discussants and those nearby. A lone airman smoked cigarette after cigarette, nervously running a hand through his hair. Another read a *Stag* magazine, although the nude photos didn't appear to interest him.

No one knew what was expected, but everyone tried to avoid an embarrassing episode rather than display anxiety or emotion of pending separation. I had not forged strong opinions of the war or its morality. As most Americans during that time, I believed South Vietnam desired a democratic future and the United States was helping to achieve that goal, but I had little knowledge of Vietnamese life or culture. News coverage of the war increasingly focused on differences between governmental statements and conditions on the ground. The reports increased my skepticism of politicians, but I did not actively oppose the war. In 1966, no one could foresee the long, bloody, and duplicitous course of U.S. involvement. Nevertheless, cracks in America's faith in its government were beginning to appear.

A monotone voice announced flight No. 243 to Saigon would load. Last-minute handshakes and embraces were exchanged, and passengers rushed to their queue.

The lines shuffled to the Pan American 707. I grabbed Keith's hand and gave Kathie a hug. It was a quick walk down the ramp to the plane. It was November 3, 1966, and I was about to embark on my yearlong tour in Vietnam overseeing a medical unit in the delta.

The aircraft had been modified to accommodate 158 military passengers. The uniformed Pan Am stewardesses politely assisted the uniformed passengers as they would civilians. What an odd way to go to war, I thought—it could almost be misconstrued with taking an exotic Southeastern Asia vacation. It reminded me of how the French rode taxis to the battle of Marne during World War I.

It felt strange to finally depart for Vietnam. Last week I was classifying *Anopheles* mosquito larvae under a dissecting microscope at Fort Sam Houston, Texas; three months earlier I treated dependent personnel in a Chicago army dispensary. Moreover, I had only graduated from medical school two years prior and was in my mid–20s. Was I capable of leading a group of doctors and corpsmen? I hoped so, and vowed to meet the challenge and to document my efforts, as within a few days I would command a Military Provincial Health Assistance Program (MILPHAP) unit in Bac Lieu.

I knew nothing could prepare me for the atrocities and primitive medical conditions I was about to face. But I was ready to help the unfortunate citizens of the province.

Becoming a doctor was in my blood. My father, Eldon, was a kindly man who graduated from medical school and married in 1929, right before the throes of the Great Depression. As a result, he struggled to develop a practice in Iowa as patients bartered with vegetables and fruits for his services.

After a couple of years, he hitched a ride to Los Angeles, an area less affected by the Depression and where he was promised a medical partnership. In 1935 he struck out on his own, opening an office a few blocks away where loyal patients followed. He loved obstetrics and delivered more than 2,000 babies, including many for family and friends. In fact, vacations and weekend events were frequently cancelled awaiting a delivery, as he had no partner and women knew he would be available throughout their pregnancy. My mother and I waited countless hours in the family car as he made evening house calls or visited the hospital.

After dinner we frequently watched 16 mm movies of surgical technique as my father prepared for an operation. I learned to gown and mask after observing him performing surgery at a local hospital or minor procedures in the office. I viewed my first autopsy at age 11 or 12 and was captivated by Axel Munthe's *San Michele* and the tragedy of Semmelweis. We'd take "vacations" to big cities as he enrolled in surgical refresher courses. He typified the family doctor of the era—compassionate and steadfast. My uncle designed a doctor's office with living quarters on the second floor, which was the Carlson Medical Building for more than 30 years. However, patients knew my father was upstairs and there was no respite from 24/7 duty, prompting our move to La Cañada a few miles distant.

As a youth, I never thought of anything but becoming a doctor. I waded through high school and Occidental College and began medical school at the University of Southern California (USC). My father was certainly happy when I chose that path, but the intellectual abilities of my classmates and the rigor of the curriculum were challenging. USC introduced me to the Los Angeles County General Hospital (LACGH), the huge clinical city that provided medical care for LA's socially and medically deprived population. I didn't know it at the time, but it would be the best training for what I'd experience in Bac Lieu.

As a freshman med student, I was intimidated by the "Great Stone Mother," as LACGH was called. The art deco cement structure was completed in 1933, one of the largest hospitals in the country—it housed nearly 2,000 beds on 20 floors, with two basements and a tunnel. (The building continues to dominate the landscape of Lincoln Heights, although the hospital has been replaced by the LAC-USC Medical Center a block away.) The patients we saw were quite diverse, most of whom were down on their luck and didn't have money for care.

In 1961, I and the other freshmen med students would trudge across the street from the medical school campus to a side entrance of the mammoth building to see patients who allowed the young students in short white coats to take clinical histories and perform physical examinations after we practiced on one another.

By the third year of medical school, I was more comfortable with the massive edifice and had explored much of the building during clinical clerkships. On medicine rotations, we took calls with the resident and intern team and were each assigned a patient to work up and follow. After completing a history and physical, and assisting with procedures, we could go home by 9:00 or 10:00 p.m. But the team remained on duty throughout the night for new admissions.

Another clinical rotation was diabetes. That's where I met Dr. Helen Martin, a legend at LA County and USC. She was one of five women to graduate from USC's medical school in 1934 and remained at that institution for more than 30 years. During World War II, most of the faculty were assigned to the 76th Evacuation hospital in Burma, while Dr. Martin and a few others shepherded the LA County Hospital and USC medical school through the war years.

She specialized in diabetes and knew many of the patients personally. Under her supervision, junior medical students admitted patients with diabetic coma (ketoacidosis) and charted their clinical progress with a flow chart. It was a multi-hour battle fighting lethal levels of blood sugar, dehydration, and deranged electrolytes. We plotted physical findings, lab values, insulin doses, and fluids throughout the night and presented the patient to Dr. Martin the next morning, a chastening experience. She contracted polio as a child and walked with a cane, which she would tap on the floor as we spoke. It was threatening—not physically, but psychologically—as one sensed the cane transmitted her approval or disapproval of our presentation. She demanded honesty and perfection. The patients were typically our age or younger with juvenile diabetes and many could not afford to purchase lifesaving insulin. Medicare and Medicaid were not signed into law until 1965 by President Johnson, and these patients had no private insurance. The county hospital was the only recourse for vast numbers of Los Angeles residents with acute or chronic diseases or trauma.

Under Dr. Martin's guidance, we learned to titrate the management of a very sick patient, a tenet of critical care medicine I utilized throughout my career. She was a master of fluid and electrolyte physiology, but her first principle was "always do what is best for the patient." She was demanding, but compassionate and sympathetic to the young physicians in training (although she both inspired and terrified us). It was medicine at its finest.

I graduated from medical school in 1964 and remained at LA County for internship followed by the first year of Ob-Gyn residency, when I witnessed further disparity among the citizens of the City of Angels. I delivered two dozen babies a night on Obstetrics. Because of poor access to care, many women received no prenatal care and developed toxemia or other medical problems of pregnancy, often accompanied by life-threatening complications of delivery. I was fortunate to be guided by senior residents and seasoned faculty whose LA County experience had exposed them to virtually every problem that could befall a mother and baby. I also beheld the results of botched abortions and untreated malignancies. It was a tremendous education but a depressing social commentary.

During the 1965 Watts riots in Los Angeles, an Ob-Gyn ward became a surgical admission unit for gunshot victims, some of whom were friends and relatives of Black employees, yielding heartbreaking encounters.

My experiences left me unsure of what path to take next in my medical career. My father had a satisfying career as a general practitioner and was pleased when I announced I would pursue obstetrics. While I enjoyed the first year of my residency, I still wasn't certain I wanted to be a "baby doctor" the rest of my life; private practice held no allure for me. LA County had awakened me to social injustice and barriers to medical care—I knew there had to be more I could do.

My graduation from medical school in 1964 coincided with increased conflict in Southeast Asia. In August, a naval engagement known as the Gulf of Tonkin incident led to a major escalation of U.S. participation in the Vietnam conflict. The gulf is bordered by the coast of North Vietnam and the Chinese Leizhou Peninsula in the South China Sea. On August 2, the USS *Maddox*, a destroyer patrolling the area, fired warning shots at three North Vietnamese torpedo boats that approached the ship. The boats launched torpedoes and fired machine guns at the *Maddox*, which responded, damaging the boats and killing four North Vietnamese sailors. The *Maddox* retreated, but a second armed contact was reported two days later, which was subsequently proven to be false. Nevertheless, these incidents resulted in massive U.S. news coverage, including a nationally televised speech by President Johnson on the evening of August 4. The U.S. Congress responded quickly, and on August 7 passed the Gulf of Tonkin Resolution allowing President Johnson to "take all necessary measures to repel any armed attack against the forces of the United States, and to prevent further aggression by the communist government of North Vietnam."

This was a crucial step of U.S. involvement in the war, and by 1966 the draft of men into military service increased substantially, raising U.S. forces in Vietnam to 385,000, and ultimately conscripting more than two million Americans until the draft was abolished in 1973. The domino theory proclaimed by Eisenhower 12 years earlier propelled U.S. policy to combat communist expansion with force.

As a physician I was subject to the draft, and with nearly one-half of my fellow 1964 USC graduates, I took the chance I would not be called and did not enroll in the

Berry Plan, which would have allowed me to defer military service until I had completed my residency. In 1966, I was finishing the first year of obstetrics-gynecology residency when I learned of my service in the U.S. Army Medical Corps. I was relieved when drafted, as it allowed me to contemplate my career options while continuing to serve.

My first stop was basic training for physicians at Fort Sam Houston, Texas, followed by assignment to a dispensary in Chicago. People told me I had it made, but my army experience was relatively boring, and I knew within months I would be deployed to Vietnam as a general medical officer (GMO) in a military medical facility.

While in basic training in Texas, I learned of new teams to aid Vietnam's civilians, termed MILPHAP. They reported to USAID (United States Agency for International Development) but remained within the military. There was a critical shortage of health resources for Vietnam's 16 million people and most doctors were assigned to the military. Less than 300 of Vietnam's 1,000 physicians were available for civilian practice. MILPHAP units were placed in Vietnam's civilian hospitals to treat citizens affected by the war and the country's many endemic diseases.

A team consisted of three physicians, a Medical Service Corps (MSC) officer, and 12 enlisted corpsmen, and was responsible to the province medicine chief to augment the hospital's meager staff. Some units were bolstered by USAID nurses, including where I was headed. The program had only been in operation a year, and more teams were planned, including those from other countries.

Civilian health care in Vietnam was a disaster, but the experience would be a huge challenge and an opportunity.

During my assignment in Chicago, I applied and was astonished to learn not only had I been accepted, but would command a MILPHAP team of doctors, nurses, and enlisted men in the Bac Lieu province hospital in the Mekong delta. Returning to Fort Sam Houston, I took courses in preventive medicine, infectious disease, and tropical medicine.

My family, especially my father, were perplexed why I volunteered for Vietnam. Confused, but supportive, he wondered what my military interlude would yield. He wasn't alone. My MILPHAP assignment generated a mixture of anticipation and anxiety. To treat victims of the war and see exotic diseases would be exciting, but I could not fathom the tumultuous year before me.

While in Texas preparing for my MILPHAP assignment, I received a letter from the doctor I would replace in Bac Lieu. He wrote:

> This is a 200-bed hospital, although we usually have more patients than beds. The facility represents the only significant treatment center for almost 300,000 civilians. The hospital is a series of tile and stone buildings built by the French in 1909. The buildings are separated by mud and a few cement walks. Most of our wards don't have electricity or running water, but there is a generator for surgery and X-ray. Dr. Vinh, a surgeon, is the Province Medicine Chief. You will be working with and for him. Another Vietnamese physician, Dr. Khoung, oversees one of the medical wards. Dr. Tot, a female doctor, works in obstetrics and the female medical ward. Lab facilities are very primitive. We live in the adjacent U.S. MACV compound that houses approximately 100 advisors to the 21st ARVN (Army of Vietnam) division. Aside from the heat and dirt, we probably have better quarters than most

Americans in Vietnam. There is a small medical library, but if you have a favorite medical text—bring it! You will also need a few sport shirts, slacks and a large fan. Most of our current team will have rotated home by your arrival. You will therefore have to orient yourself to the hospital. GOOD LUCK!

I reread the letter several times during the flight that took me to Alaska and Japan before finally landing in Saigon. My Vietnam adventure was about to begin.

Chapter Sources

Michael R. Cousineau and Robert E. Tranquada. "Crisis and Commitment: 150 Years of Service by Los Angeles County Public Hospitals." *American Journal of Public Health* 97, no. 4 (2007): 606–15.

Sarah Lifton. *Keck School of Medicine and the University of Southern California: Trials and Transformation.* Old Saybrook, CT: Greenwich, 2004.

Axel Munthe. *The Story of San Michele.* New York: E. P. Dutton, 1929.

Morton Thompson. *The Cry and the Covenant.* New York: Buccaneer Books, 1949.

2

Saigon

Pearl of the Orient

On the final leg of our journey, the cabin's atmosphere changed dramatically. Mainland China was visible at dawn below our starboard wing—the Red Dragon appeared peaceful from 30,000 feet. But now my fellow passengers fidgeted, cigarettes were lit, and conversation became more animated. Others retreated silently to their thoughts. I experienced gastric irritability coupled with a dry mouth that accompanies anxiety. I reassured myself my Vietnam experience would be benign compared to most of those on board. But I also knew I was flying into a war zone; anything could happen. This realization confronted me as I looked at the ocean below. I yawned and my mouth was dry as I recalled Barnaby Conrad's description of matadors in *Gates of Fear*: if a matador can spit before a corrida, he is either very brave or very foolish.

A smoky pall partially obscured our view of Saigon, Pearl of the Orient, as it was called. On our final approach, we crossed a river where small boats were busily transporting matériel from ships along the wharf. Tan Son Nhut had become one of the busiest airports in the world. Our Boeing landed and taxied past rows of military and civilian aircraft of all varieties, escorted by an air police jeep brandishing a machine gun. The cabin door opened to sultry heat. My first sight was an Asian girl wearing black pajamas covered by a loose-fitting sheath of white silk and a pair of spiked heels. I had no time to savor the view, as I was pushed down the gangway by my fellow passengers. It was also the first of many encounters of rampant racism. I cringed as an SP4 (Specialist 4) exclaimed from the rear of the line, "Jesus, look at all the slope-heads … a lot of gooks." A group of Vietnamese were squatting behind a barricade adjacent to the ramp.

The term "gook" originated in the 1890s and referred to Filipinos during the Spanish-American War. Gook and other derogatory terms, such as wog, chink, nip, or slope-head, dehumanize a group of people. The average American soldier in Vietnam was 19 years old, with scant prior contact with Asians, called "Orientals" at that time, another ethnic slur. The terms gook and slope-head were also applied to the 35,000 Asian American soldiers who fought in Vietnam. The racism went beyond name-calling, as these men often encountered poor or delayed medical care following battle injury, and incidents were documented when they were fired upon by their comrades, although the Viet Cong specifically targeted Asian soldiers. Filipino sailors were relegated to serve as stewards on navy vessels. Despite these hardships, four Medal of

Honor awards were given posthumously to Asian American soldiers. President Truman integrated the military two decades earlier, but the process was far from complete.

Ton Son Nhut's terminal was a huge open-air building with large fans that battled flies and heat. Although humid, the temperature was bearable.

After learning I was not part of a group of doctors bound for military installations, I waited for a car to transport me to Military Assistance Command, Vietnam (MACV) headquarters. An army sedan ultimately arrived, and I was treated to a hair-raising ride through Saigon by an overzealous SP5 driver. The roads teemed with all manner of vehicles—bicycles, cyclos, scooters, dogcarts, cars, buses, trucks, and modes of transport that defied description, none of which were given quarter by my driver. "You can't let these gooks bluff you," he exclaimed with bravado, narrowly missing an old man on a bicycle. We eventually stopped in front of a large, white building rimmed by 50-gallon drums filled with cement and surrounded by a barbed wire fence. A military police officer behind a guard post saluted and smiled as I dragged my gear through the gate. I regretted the thoroughness of my packing, especially several heavy medical books.

The building was formerly a hospital and more recently a hotel. I was relieved to see two familiar faces in the lobby—Dick Muir and Boyd Mullholand, both of whom shared MILPHAP course work with me in Texas.

A plaque in the lobby indicated the building was named for Major Koelper, killed during a terrorist attack. The compound consisted of two major structures—a billet, plus offices and classrooms. A coffin-sized elevator was in the main building but was not operational most of the time. Water was provided twice a day. Even with this limited schedule, the archaic plumbing frequently rebelled with no hot or running water. I was assigned a room on the 6th floor, a chamber approximately 10-by-10 feet, with a set of bunk beds and a dresser, topped by whiskey bottles filled with potable water replaced daily by Vietnamese maids. The walls were a bilious green, crisscrossed with a mass of exposed wiring and pipes. Small lizards on the ceiling defied gravity. In the center of the room an overhead fan turned slowly. Each room had a small closet, plus an adjoining bathroom with shower where an open hole in the floor provided drainage. The fuse box and light switches were placed next to the hot- and cold-water valves. To avoid electrocution, one stood in the bedroom and reached across the wet floor to the opposite wall. The rooms cost 25 piastres a day—at 118 piastres to a U.S. dollar, a very reasonable rate—although the accommodations were spartan.

The second building was air-conditioned, with classrooms and offices. Sandbags had been placed at all entrances and windows were taped to prevent shattering in case of enemy ordnance. A small, third structure included the mailroom, a tiny post exchange military store (PX), and a snack bar.

After a supper of canned chili laced with Tabasco sauce and an overcooked hamburger, the three exhausted MILPHAP doctors climbed the staircase to our floors and were in bed by 8:00 p.m.

The next day was Sunday and briefings were curtailed. I was beginning to make sense of the military alphabet soup: MACV was Military Assistance Command Vietnam—which directed all military aspects of American activity. MACV was led by General William Westmoreland, and was preceded by MAAG, or Military

Assistance Advisory Group, which began operation in 1956. MACV had jurisdiction over USARV, or United States Army Vietnam. ARVN—Army of the Republic of Vietnam—was the Vietnamese military. MACV's primary responsibility was command and to provide advisory teams for ARVN. In Bac Lieu, the advisors for the 21st ARVN division and MILPHAP's quarters were housed in the MACV compound.

A master sergeant gave a lecture entitled "How to Stay Alive in Saigon," quoting gory details of recent terrorist bombings of officer quarters and bus stops, as well as knifings in movies, mines in a floating restaurant, and taxicab kidnappings. We learned a favorite Viet Cong terrorist technique was to detonate a mine on a motor scooter or rickshaw across from a U.S. billet or bus stop. A second would be detonated several seconds later, increasing the number of casualties.

A private first class (PFC) carried several round metal objects to the lectern. Pointing to the items, the sergeant explained: "These, gentlemen, are DH-10 claymore mines. The claymore is the workhorse of Viet Cong mines and has an effective casualty radius of 16 to 20 meters." The devices were the size of an automobile wheel rim and painted a dull black.

He continued, "These are easily concealed and can be placed where you'd never guess—in piles of manure, on trees, or in potholes." He picked up a small doll and added, "Our devious friends also fabricate a variety of innocent appearing items which are passed to GIs. This doll contains enough explosives to kill everyone in this room. We caught it in the mail—a soldier had sent it to his girlfriend in the states as a souvenir. Cigarette lighters, ball-point pens, match boxes, and other trinkets can also be used as anti-personnel weapons. So, the next time you go to your favorite club on Tu Do Street, don't lay your lighter on the bar."

Putting his notes aside, the sergeant concluded, "I have a few hints for you: Don't eat on the local economy if you can help it. Stay away from the girls unless you want a dose of the clap or worse, and don't buy from black market street vendors. You can probably get it cheaper at the PX. Always travel in groups of two or more. And, by the way, there is an 11:00 p.m. curfew in Saigon. Good morning, gentlemen."

Despite warnings, Dick, Boyd, and I decided to explore the city. It was 10:00 a.m., but the temperature had reached 98 degrees and we were soaked with sweat. We pondered our mode of transportation. The government furnished buses with color-coded route signs and schedules. They were safe and the windows enclosed with mesh. But they were slow and unpredictable. You could hitch a ride on one of the many motor scooters, but they were exposed during the frequent rains. There were also foot-operated cyclopeds, or cyclos, which were basically an easy chair in front of a bike. Though they were designed for one passenger, two or three Vietnamese frequently crowded the seat. Bikes were slow and at the mercy of the maddening traffic. One could walk, although sidewalk vendors made it a perilous gauntlet. In the end, we settled on a taxi, which was most convenient and only cost 25 piastres for the trip downtown.

Saigon was home to more than 1.5 million people, but its area was no larger than a U.S. city of 50,000 to 100,000 population. The Chinese section was Cholon, where the main PX was located. After a tour of Saigon and the Cholon PX, we arrived at the Brinks, a billet for field grade (major and above) officers. The top floor featured a bar

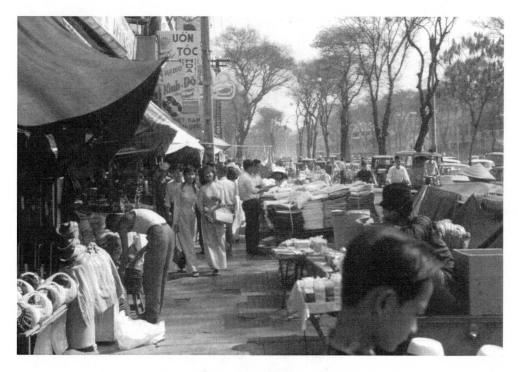

Saigon sidewalk black-market vendors.

and one of the best restaurants in the city. Drinks were strong and cheap, with lively entertainment. Adjacent to the bar, a Vietnamese quintet belted out U.S. standards, as stewards loaded the projector for the evening's film. The food was good, and the fresh pineapple and other salad items were particularly appetizing. I was surprised to see many American women in cocktail dresses.

After dinner we checked out Tu Do Street. This locale was famous for its many bars, which were hot, dank, and expensive. Young girls lounged outside establishments with names like Blue Angel, Texas Bar, and Bunny Club, all designed to lure GIs inside. A local beer called 33, or "ba muoi ba," cost 100 piastres. At the bar or a table, tea girls made their appearance. Their presence cost an additional 150–250 piastres every 10 minutes. Patrons were frequently encouraged to buy them tea and order more drinks. The girls appeared friendly and permitted GIs amazing liberties to be fondled, but they were emotionally cold and could barely be understood, except to urge purchase of more drinks. The girls appeared to be 17 or 18 years old, although management insisted they were at least 21. I was told the girls received 50 percent of profit for each round of drinks, although another source said their commission was much smaller. You could dance with them if you continued to buy. The rounds kept coming until the girl was dismissed. In the event more intimate entertainment was desired, the club's "mamason" was contacted and bargaining continued. We drank a 33 and returned to Koepler by cab.

Chapter Sources

Barnaby Conrad. *Gates of Fear.* New York: Bonanza Books, 1957.

3

Getting Familiar

Our early days were filled with briefings. A major described air operations and military logistics. The United States began the big buildup in 1964, and the 7th Air Force was created. By early 1966, the in-country strike force included more than 300 U.S. Air Force aircraft, 300 U.S. Navy and marine planes, and 145 Vietnamese. More than 80,000 sorties had been flown during the first six months of 1966.

Not all the briefings told the full story. In fact, we were completely misled by the briefing on defoliation missions by U.S. aircraft. The result was destroyed vegetation, which meant loss of cover for Viet Cong troops and their equipment. Approximately two to three weeks after spraying a jungle or forested region, leaves and other superficial growth would be shed, exposing the area. Other chemicals were used to destroy Viet Cong rice paddies, denying the enemy potential food stores and funds. The briefing officer lauded the effectiveness of these activities and told us of plans to expand the program. He said the chemicals were safe and like those employed for American farming. With complete air superiority, spraying of chemicals proceeded at will, "without risk." He asserted defoliation was one of the most important activities of the war effort.

In addition to aerial spraying, we learned planes and helicopters were constantly in flight over major cities and military installations, assisted by radio communication and radar to report and monitor enemy activities. Night missions carried flares to light suspect areas, and reconnaissance missions equipped with infrared monitors could create aerial maps in flight, as well as photograph and process films. Viet Cong campfires otherwise not visible in the jungle were detected. The infrared sensors were able to identify a vehicle that hadn't been operated for several hours, even if stored in a shed.

The United States initiated defoliation missions in 1961 under President Kennedy, who authorized the first aerial spraying. The program was termed Operation Ranch Hand and was part of an overall chemical warfare activity, Operation Trail Dust, which continued for 10 years. Chemicals were supplied by the Dow and Monsanto companies, and included both herbicides and defoliants, contaminated by a highly toxic material, dioxin. The amount of dioxin and its effects weren't initially known, but were eventually proven to be extremely toxic. In addition, the concentration of chemicals used in Vietnam was far greater than agricultural use, and many regions received multiple applications. More than 20 million gallons of defoliants and herbicides were applied to five million acres of forests and jungles and 500,000 acres of crops. Two-thirds of all Vietnamese hamlets were affected, exposing 4.8 million civilians.

Spraying involved the U.S. Air Force with C-123 cargo planes equipped with 1,000-gallon tanks. A single plane could spray a swath 80 meters wide and 16 km long in four to five minutes. Typically, several planes flew abreast, exposing a wider area of distribution. At least 20,000 sorties were flown during the 10 years of operation. Several cocktails of chemicals were employed for forest or crop applications. The most common combination was "Agent Orange," which utilized two agents, plus the dioxin contamination. The name was based on the colored stripes of the 55-gallon drums. Other mixtures included Agent White and Agent Blue. Since the materials were thought to be safe, no special precautions, such as use of protective gloves, aprons, or coveralls, were taken by those handling the chemicals, flight crews, or others. In addition to handlers, hundreds of thousands of ground personnel were exposed.

Years later, I learned the information presented at the briefing on chemicals was false: defoliation did involve risk, caused great harm, and led to the death of thousands, including one of my Bac Lieu colleagues.

Beginning 1964, the Federation of American Scientists objected to the program. The American Association for the Advancement of Science (AAAS) passed a resolution to study the program and in 1967 urged the Department of Defense to halt use of herbicides. This coincided with a petition, which was signed by 17 Nobel laureates and 5,000 scientists, to immediately terminate the program. The U.S. administration ignored the request. Philosopher and peace advocate Bertrand Russell claimed the United States was using carcinogenic herbicides in Vietnam. The response was to brand the elderly Russell senile. But protests continued and the program was ultimately abandoned in the early 1970s.

Health effects, including genetic defects from contaminated soil, continue to be studied among U.S. veterans as well as Vietnamese. Exposure has been linked to multiple diseases, including amyloidosis, leukemias, lymphomas, type 2 diabetes, ischemic heart disease, multiple myeloma, Parkinson's disease, various neuropathies, porphyria, lung and other respiratory malignancies, prostate cancer, and soft tissue tumors. Several hundred thousand American and Vietnamese premature deaths have resulted from this program.

We also received a counterinsurgency (CI) operation briefing. CI was defined as any program to counter or oppose the Viet Cong. The officer stated CI programs were currently effective, but warned they would fail if the government falls or if there's an erosion of popular opinion. The Saigon government's prestige was buoyed by helping villages and hamlets formerly under Viet Cong control. But the vacuum must be filled with projects to aid the village. The speaker said these activities were evolving, as many villagers knew little of the Saigon government except for taxes and Viet Cong propaganda. During the prior Diem regime, great progress in CI was touted, but most claims were false. The officer said CI activities had been expanded and were more effective under the current government but reminded us that nation building at the local level is difficult, slow, and unrewarding work. That said, he noted it's as important as military operations—perhaps more so. As he spoke, I wondered how successful these efforts would become. Most of the audience seemed unimpressed with the speaker's claims.

USAID had developed multiple projects to aid VN citizens, including public health. MILPHAP was one example, and USAID provided hospitals with medical equipment and supplies, although the Vietnam Ministry of Health (MOH) controlled distribution. USAID also furnished agricultural, economic, and industrial support.

The briefing ended with a description of MACV's role advising and training Vietnam forces. Most of the officers in the room would be advisors, either in military roles or civilian activities, such as MILPHAP. Vietnamese military bases were unique, as they were the only training facilities operating under combat conditions.

The next day featured even more briefings. While some of the information was helpful, I was anxious to see things for myself. But it was helpful to learn about the surroundings that would be my home for the next year.

In the mid–1960s the population of South Vietnam was approximately 16 million with four military regions or corps, containing 43 provinces, roughly equivalent to states. But a province is roughly the size of a large U.S. county. The I Corps began at the demilitarized zone in the North, and IV Corps included the southernmost portion of the country and the Mekong Delta. There was a corresponding military sector for each province. Provinces were further partitioned into 252 districts, 2,550 villages, and more than 8,000 hamlets—the smallest unit of political and geographic organization, with 100 inhabitants or less. Many hamlets were dramatically altered by the war, creating two million refugees and severe inflation. The cost of living had increased 75 percent in one year, complicating life for citizens, most of whom were peasants.

Provinces were governed by province chiefs and councils once elected, but in 1966, appointed by the military. Local military units were the regional forces (RF) or popular forces (PF). RF-PF were full-time volunteer small combat elements, operating at the village or hamlet level. "Ruff-Puff" were more active fighters than one might imagine and included more personnel than ARVN's total manpower. In 1966, RF-PF accounted for more killed or captured Viet Cong than any other group. Unfortunately, the local forces were poorly trained and equipped and suffered many casualties. The RF-PF provided security to hamlets, but often confiscated food and lodging, negating their potential psychological advantages.

The officer concluded his remarks emphasizing the Vietnamese military was making consistent progress. Since 1962, allied forces had killed or captured more than 26,000 enemy. The Viet Cong's strength was estimated to be 280,000. "Of course," the officer added, "to this must be added local enlistments and those from North Vietnam." The Lao Dong party in North Vietnam ultimately controlled all enemy operations, but day-to-day conduct of the war was often fought by the Viet Cong, especially in the delta. It was incongruent, I thought to myself: If we've been making constant progress, why are the official reports so different from those of U.S. war correspondents?

On the final day of briefings, we were escorted downtown to USAID headquarters to meet Colonel William Moncrief, senior advisor and second in command to

General Humphries, Chief of USAID in Vietnam. Moncrief was an army physician on loan to USAID. A trim, energetic man with graying crew-cut hair, he wore an open white shirt and light gray slacks, and did most of the talking, but listened intently to our questions. I was impressed by his easy-going professionalism.

"I know you boys have been briefed to death at Koelper, so I won't try to tell you everything," he began. "Here's what you need to know: MILPHAP teams are a permanent, continuing public health program. The project is new, but there are more than 20 teams, with more on the way. Your job is to provide and improve civilian medical care, and to expand hospital facilities and rural public health. In Saigon, we're trying to upgrade training of medical personnel, and the country's health facilities. Your task is in the provinces—where the action is. It's a big job and you'll encounter many frustrations—if you don't, you won't be doing your job."

Under USAID, civilian medical programs in Vietnam expanded rapidly in the 1960s, including PHAP. The first MILPHAP team was initiated November 1965, in Can Tho. By 1970, teams were in 30 provincial hospitals, with Army, Navy and Air Force units, plus New Zealand, Iran, South Korea, Spain, and other countries. Teams were reorganized in 1969 to provide more surgical expertise, because of escalation of the war and greater civilian casualties.

Major General William H. Moncrief, Jr., was a career military medical officer, son of a famed army colonel. Moncrief attended Emory University School of Medicine, followed by training in surgery and thoracic-cardiovascular surgery. His 31 years of military service included World War II, Korea, and Vietnam. In 1966, he was assigned to the State Department to oversee civilian health for Vietnam, when I met him. During his illustrious career, he served as commanding officer of Brooke General Hospital and the Letterman and Walter Reed Army Medical centers, and was the recipient of numerous awards.

As an afterthought, Moncrief added, "Another thing: don't confuse MILPHAP with MEDCAP [Medical Civic Action Program]. MEDCAP is a mobile setup strictly outpatient, usually a one-time visit in rural areas. It's designed as a psy-war program, under supervision of medical officers, but usually run by corpsmen. Although military commanders love MEDCAPs, your mission is more permanent and important. MILPHAP teams are exempted from MEDCAP missions. Remember, your job is to provide permanent, continuous medical care. You'll be the guest of the medicine chief of the provincial hospital. He has the last word and is the chief provincial health officer. Working with him will require a great deal of skill and tact."

The colonel handed us manila folders and we were ushered to a conference room to read our reports. Boyd's dealt with Quang Ngai. Dick had been assigned to Pleiku. I picked through the Bac Lieu file and selected a mimeographed sheet titled "Physical Characteristics and History of Bac Lieu Province." It read:

> Bac Lieu is 165 km south of Saigon, in the lower Mekong Delta of IV Corps. The province's area is 2,000 square kilometers and is a flat, alluvial plain. It is bordered on the west by An Xuyen, on the north and northeast by Chuong Thien and Ba Xuyen provinces, and to the south by the South China Sea. The elevation of Bac Lieu ranges from sea level to 4 meters above mean high tide.
>
> The shore consists of dense mangrove forests, extending 100 meters to 6 kilometers inland.

These mangrove swamps serve as a refuge for insurgents. Off-shore the sand and mud flats extend up to three kilometers. During the spring and summer, the rice fields are flooded and 70% of the region is covered with water.

The population of Bac Lieu is approximately 280,000, of whom 80,000 are controlled or affected by the Viet Cong. At least 85% of the people are farmers. Rice is the major crop, although many harvest salt during the dry season, together with grapes, cabbage, coconuts, and pineapples. Buffalo, ducks, pigs, and other livestock are also raised. Bac Lieu is known for its fish and sea food. There is little industry, but Bac Lieu is considered one of the richest agricultural provinces in the delta.

Buddhism is the dominant religion; approximately 80–90% are Buddhist, whereas 3–5% are Catholic, and less than 1% are Protestant. Caodai, formerly an important political force, make up 2% to 6% of the population. The Hoa Hoa comprise less than 1%.

Dick looked up and exclaimed, "Pleiku ran out of penicillin two months ago!" Boyd added, "My hospital is nearly out of IV fluids—boy, this is going to be quite a year."

I continued reading my report.

The term "Bac Lieu" is a product of Vietnamese mispronunciation of "Po Lieu," meaning fish crop, which was given by the Chinese several centuries ago. Little history is known until the French rule. The country was probably originally occupied by Cambodians, although there was a Chinese immigration near the end of the 17th century. This was followed by an influx of people from what is now central and northern Vietnam. King Tu Duo settled the region and established the province in 1847. In 1882 the province was reorganized by the French into four districts which are similar to the current units: Vinh Loi (Bac Lieu), with a population of 80,000; Vinh Chau, with 52,000; Gia Rai, with 86,000; and Phuouc Long, containing 40,000 people. Of the 158 hamlets, 86 are controlled by the Saigon government, 50 are contested, and 62 are under Viet Cong control.

I was anxious to read about the hospital but found little on the topic. Instead, a typed page described the Bac Lieu climate:

The region experiences two distinct weather seasons. The dry season, from October to April, and the wet season from May to September. The monsoons come from the southwest, the Gulf of Thailand. It is said the word "monsoon" is derived from an ancient term for "big wind." During the dry season 5 or more inches of rain occur, whereas up to 50 inches falls during the wet season. Temperatures range from 75 to 95 degrees Fahrenheit, although extremes above 125 Fahrenheit have been measured.

I finally found a folder about the hospital:

Bac Lieu provincial hospital was constructed by the French in 1909. It is classified as a 210-bed institution, although the daily census is 250 or more patients. Dr. Nguyen Tu Vinh, a surgeon, has been the Medicine Chief since the early 1960s.

Other sections of the report described an X-ray machine that was frequently inoperative. Delivery of medications was typically five months late. A USAID nurse described her inability to visit some of the wards because of mud. Several large animals used the hospital grounds for pasture, and none of the windows had glass or screens. Electricity was intermittent and provided by a diesel generator.

Undeterred, we finished reading and decided to have dinner at the Brinks BOQ (Bachelor Officers' Quarters). After dinner, I bid my comrades adieu and retreated to the bar. A perspiring husky fellow in a Hawaiian shirt sat down beside me and ordered a double bourbon. "Sorry," he exclaimed, as he adjusted his barstool, "I don't think I've seen you before—new in country?"

"I arrived last Saturday," I said.

"Civilian or military?"

"Military," I admitted, "I'm headed to the delta."

Minutes passed and we ordered more drinks. It was obvious he wanted to talk. He pulled a handkerchief and blew his nose noisily, "Damn sinuses; nothing seems to help." Looking at me he continued, "I'm civilian. I work at Tan Son Nhut in processing."

I was puzzled, "Processing?"

"Yes…. Sooner or later, everyone comes to Tan Son Nhut. We take care of the boys who leave the country in steel boxes—I'm with the mortuary service." My mind returned to medical school and the pervasive odor of formaldehyde during gross anatomy class—everyone had a runny nose. No wonder he has sinus trouble. Two officers sitting next to him frowned and moved away.

He was amused I was not offended by his statement but nodded knowingly when I told him I was a doctor. He continued, "All remains are processed through our facility. We have a No. 2 priority for aircraft leaving Vietnam. And we need it—this hot weather is terrible for our business. During busy periods we sometimes work around the clock. All killed troops are sent out of the country—back to the States. No one stays here. I guess families want 'em home, and we sure send enough back. Because of the heat and delays en route, we must embalm all remains before they leave the airfield." He turned to ask me how many I thought they processed in a month. I guessed 40 or 50.

"Nope," he added. "We handle a minimum of 250 bodies a month—sometimes we do more than 30 a day. The trauma is pretty awful."

It was a difficult figure to wrap my head around. But by 1967, monthly deaths were consistently greater than 400, and usually twice that amount. Total U.S. casualties for the war exceeded 58,000, of which approximately 10,000 were not directly related to enemy action.

I couldn't take much more, although he was anxious to talk. I made my excuses and walked to the MACV compound in a somber mood. High above, planes dropped flares that slowly descended to earth, suspended by tiny parachutes like a 4th of July experience. What a war, I thought.

The next day, Dick, Boyd, and I played hooky, as briefings concerned combat operations. We took a cab to a wharf where the German hospital ship *Helgoland* was moored. Germany was neutral but provided humanitarian aid as did Canada and other countries. Dr. Wagner, a handsome young German physician, bade us aboard and gave us a tour of the beautiful 150-bed floating treatment center. We saw few patients. Unfortunately, the ship did not train Vietnamese health workers, or educate the populace on basic sanitation or hygiene. Local citizens regarded the ship as a curiosity. Dr. Wagner and his colleagues were frustrated they couldn't do more to help the people. The ship was ultimately moved to Da Nang where for several years it served a larger role in its mission of mercy.

My final day in Saigon was spent arranging transport to Bac Lieu. I collected my issued goods, which included a .45 pistol and holster that never saw action, three sets of jungle fatigues, jungle boots, and a helmet. I knew this was my last day before things would get incredibly real.

Chapter Sources

James H. Dwyer and Dieter Flesch-Janys. "Agent Orange in Vietnam." *American Journal of Public Health* 85, no. 4 (1995): 476–8.

National Academies of Sciences, Engineering, and Medicine. *Veterans and Agent Orange: Update 11 (2018).* Washington, D.C.: National Academies Press, 2018. https://doi.org/10.17226/25137.

Arnold Schecter, Le Cao Dai, Le Thu Thuy, et al. "Agent Orange and the Vietnamese: The persistence of elevated dioxin levels in human tissues." *American Journal of Public Health* 85, no. 4 (1995): 516–22.

Jeanne M. Stellman and Steven D. Stellman. "Agent Orange During the Vietnam War: The Lingering Issue of the Civilian and Military Health Impact." *American Journal of Public Health* 108, no. 6 (2018): 726–28.

Alvin L. Young and Paul F. Cecil, Jr., "Agent Orange Exposure and Attributed Health Effects in Vietnam Veterans." *Military Medicine* 176, no. 7 (2011): 29–34.

Neil Spurgeon. "Medical Assistance to Vietnamese Civilians." Chap. 13 in *Medical Support of the U.S. Army in Vietnam 1965–70.* Washington, D.C.: U.S. Government Printing Office, 1973.

William H. Moncrief Jr., Major General, U.S. Army (Ret.). Obituary. *Washington Post*, May 6, 2012.

4

Welcome to Bac Lieu

On the morning of our departure, Dick, Boyd, and I loaded our gear into a taxi and drove to Ton Son Nhut. I sat on my duffle bag, guarding our goods as they entered the dispatch office. Dick emerged a few minutes later with bad news. "Sorry, there are no flights to Bac Lieu for three days," he said. I went to the office and pleaded with the officer. "Vung Tau is the best I can do," he suggested. I had no idea where Vung Tau was, but accepted his offer, and spent several hours waiting to be called as others departed.

Vung Tau was a picturesque seaside resort that had become a huge supply depot and the site of the new 36 Evacuation hospital. In the dispensary I luckily found a USC classmate, Lou Cohen, who arranged a ride to Bac Lieu the next day and overnight quarters at the "Bac Si barracks."

Everyone in Vung Tau had a tape recorder and Joan Baez, Barbra Streisand, and the Beatles were the craze. Expensive Japanese machines were purchased at the PX and dutifully set up in quarters. Unfortunately, the local electricity was 50 cycle, which affected the tapes. One rendition of a Beatles song sounded from outer space.

The morning flight from Vung Tau to Bac Lieu on a Caribou, or 'bou, was a milk run with six stops, allowing me to appreciate delta scenery, which resembled a flooded Iowa—flat, with many small farms connected by canals and streams filled with brown water and few roads.

Eventually we came to Bac Lieu. The plane touched the tarmac, throwing spray on the windows as it traversed puddles. The pilot reversed the propellers' pitch and we abruptly came to a stop. Walking aft, the crew chief raised the fuselage door. "Bac Lieu—last stop," he shouted over the roar of the engines. I scrambled off as the chief threw out my luggage. A PFC loaded my goods into a dusty pick-up truck. A sign proclaimed: *"Bac Lieu International Airport. Runway 1700, Elevation: 2' above sea level dry season, 2' below sea level wet season. Home of 21st Division Paddy Rats."*

The airfield field was 2 km from the city. Driving along the paddies we passed a group of boys with a water buffalo who waved, yelling, "OK, Number One." Soon we came to the MACV compound, a series of aging cement buildings with tile roofs. The driver pointed to a building, "That's ADMIN," he said. "They'll get you settled."

A sergeant asked me to wait as he picked up a telephone, "We've got your new doc here—yeah. You'd better come soon—he looks a little lost."

First Lt. Donald Robinson, my MSC officer, stepped inside, exclaiming, "I'm sure glad to see you—we didn't know if you were coming. Let's get your gear. You

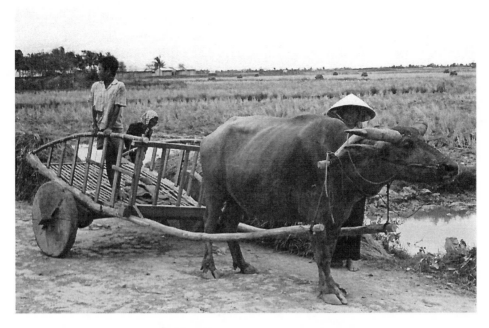

Boys and water buffalo on road to Bac Lieu.

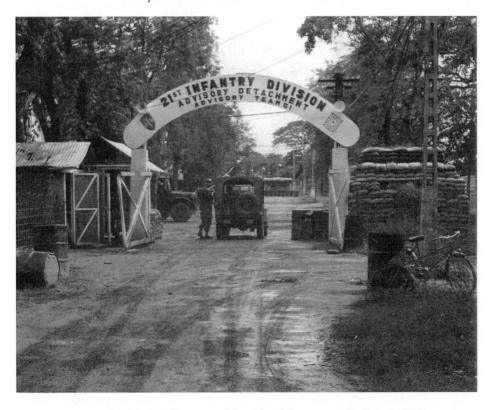

Entrance to MACV Compound Bac Lieu (photograph R. Brittis, MD).

can bunk with me." A thin, bespectacled, amiable fellow in tropical fatigues and baseball cap, Don explained he arrived a few weeks earlier. It wasn't clear when other members would come. Only four corpsmen were currently on site. We dragged my gear down the wooden walkways separating hooches. A hooch was approximately 9-by-10 feet, with two beds covered with mosquito netting, a small desk, "hot boxes" with light bulbs to prevent mildew, two chairs, and another locker. Our hooch also had a small refrigerator intended for plasma and blood but filled with beer and fresh fruit. The sides of the hooches were screened with overlapping boards to divert the rain. Walkways led to the latrine and other buildings. The term "hooch" was a recent military argot in the delta for army quarters patterned after civilian huts, although the word's origin may predate Vietnam.

Don looked at his watch. "It's about lunch time. We'll take a tour later." It began to rain as we headed to the mess hall, joined by several officers in tropical fatigues.

"Not spaghetti again!" moaned a handsome captain at a nearby table. "I'm going back to the Green Berets—at least we had decent chow." Seeing me, he extended a hand, "Hi, I'm Tom Needham—welcome to Bac Lieu. Have a seat."

A few minutes later three young women in spotless white nurse uniforms entered the mess hall with a tanned, smiling man of average height in his 40s wearing a white short-sleeved shirt. Don leaned over and whispered, "Those are the USAID nurses and Doc Owen. Come, I'll introduce you."

Nurses contracted for a year or more of VN duty with USAID, which was created by the Foreign Assistance Act of 1961 by President Kennedy. They were given a

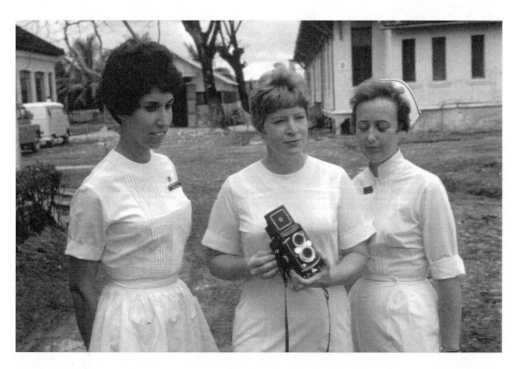

USAID Nurses Mariana Hartmann, Linda DeWolfe, and Joan Schubert in front of hospital (not shown is Pat Krebsbach).

course in Vietnamese language and served in provincial hospitals and public health facilities.

"Girls," announced Don, "this is Captain Carlson, our new MOC."

"Dick," I interjected, "Glad to meet you."

A red-haired girl sitting next to Doctor Owen smiled at me, "Hi—I'm Linda DeWolfe. This is Mariana Hartmann," pointing to a brunette next to her, "and that is Pat Krebsbach," a blond at the end of the table. "Our chief nurse, Joan Schubert, is on R&R. She'll be back next week. Oops, I almost forgot, this is Doctor Owen."

"Call me Bill," grinned Owen, as we shook hands over a plate of spaghetti. "Have you seen the hospital yet?"

"No, I just arrived," I said.

"What's your specialty?"

"Well, I was an Ob-Gyn resident before I was drafted. The army now calls me a preventive medicine officer."

Linda and Owen exchanged winks. "How do you like pediatrics?" Linda asked.

"All right, I guess." I stammered.

Linda smiled, "We've got plenty for you."

Bill Owen was a general practitioner from St. Ansgar, a small town in Iowa, and one of the volunteer physicians in the Project Vietnam program sponsored by the American Medical Association (AMA) and USAID. Physicians spent two months in province hospitals working alongside Vietnamese doctors and MILP-HAP teams. The People-to-People Foundation developed a pilot program to bring volunteer physicians for two-month intervals to work in Vietnam's provinces. The program began in 1965 and the AMA assumed management in 1966 as Volunteer Physicians for Vietnam (VPVN). During its seven-year life, 774 VPVN physicians served 1029 two-month tours in 31 of Vietnam's 43 provinces. Approximately 18 percent of physicians did repeat tours, and many returned for longer commitments. Physicians were given $10 a day compensation, with airfare and a $50,000 all-risk life insurance policy, plus assistance with passports and immunizations. Medical specialists, surgeons, and family or general practice physicians served. The AMA doctors were appalled by the primitive state of Vietnamese medical care, training, and facilities, but toiled long hours, often seeing 100 patients a day. Despite war, no serious casualties occurred during the program. There were complaints, but 98 percent of doctors said it was a positive major life experience. Physicians such as Bill Owen were invaluable to our efforts and the experience had a profound impact on their lives.

"I don't know what my partner's going to do back home until I return—but here I am," admitted Owen. "I'm sure glad I came—you'll see why once you've been around the hospital."

After lunch the girls drove Bill Owen home. Slamming the jeep's door, Bill said, "Siesta time—the hospital is closed until 2:00 p.m."

That afternoon I viewed the facility in which I would spend countless hours the coming year. Although I had read of the hospital, the sight of the crumbling buildings and unkempt grounds was overwhelming. It was immediately behind the MACV compound via a gate manned by a sentry. Leading the way, Don warned,

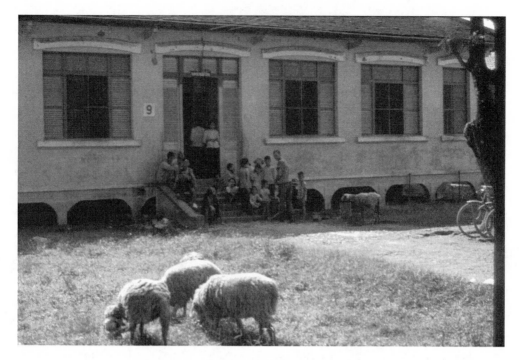

Sheep grazing on Bac Lieu hospital grounds.

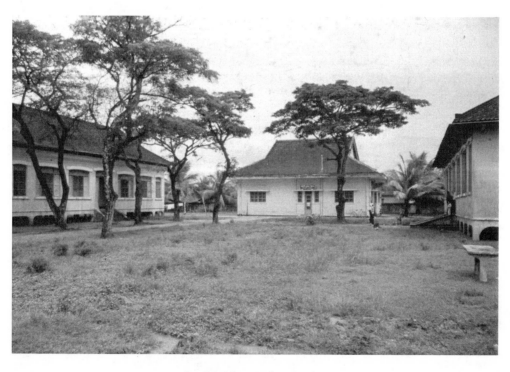

Bac Lieu hospital grounds.

"Look out for the puddles, some are nearly a foot deep." We beheld a series of yellowed cement structures, windows without screens, and crumbling tile roofs. Two or three cows and a few sheep grazed between the buildings. In front of the hospital a weathered sign proclaimed: "Phan Dinh Phung—Benh Vien."

"Phan Ding Phung," said Don, "is the name of the hospital. 'Benh Vien' means 'House of the Sick.'"

A pedicab stopped behind me as I looked at the sign, discharging a woman clutching a child. The driver grinned and mocked a salute. "Chao, Bac Si," he said as he peddled the vehicle behind me.

I looked at Don, "What did he call me?"

"'Chao' is their greeting—like, you know—hello. 'Bac Si' means 'doctor.'"

"But how did he know I was a doctor?"

"Believe me, they know. The day Doc Owen arrived he took a walk downtown and everyone knew who he was and called him Bac Si—some even used his name: Bac Si Owen."

Don pointed to a large building in front of us with plaster falling off in huge flakes. "That's the administration building—pharmacy is in the back, as well as Vinh's office." Several barefoot children ran after us and grabbed our hands as we walked. "Don't mind them, some are patients," added Don, "others live around here or belong to hospital workers."

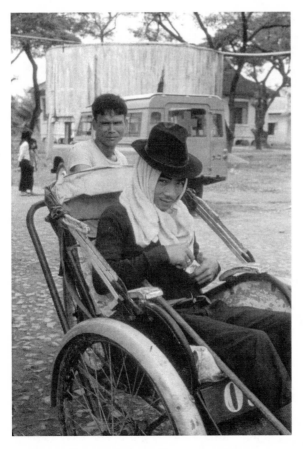

Cyclo delivering patient to hospital.

We continued walking as Don pointed out Maternity and the Emergency Room (ER). "Trai 10" was inscribed above one of the doors. As we neared the building two goats ran through the doorway and jumped over the steps. We entered a large room, vacant except for a scaffold, a few paint buckets, and a pile of rubbish in the corner. "This will be our new ER," explained my guide, as he led me through a short hall to a smaller room with a bed, table, and chair. "We currently use this cubbyhole for our night calls."

Outside, a diesel engine protested as it was started. "That's the generator—they must be getting ready for a surgery," Don added.

We passed the surgical suite

that was constructed by USAID in 1962. There were two operating rooms, although only one was used for surgery. The other housed an antique X-ray machine.

"Does the X-ray work?" I asked.

"After a fashion—Doc Owen uses it to fluoroscope fractures and bullets. We've got chemicals and film, but nobody has tried to take any pictures. Our regular X-ray machine has broken down."

Owen was scrubbing when we entered. "Hernia," he said, gesturing to the operating table where a young man was being prepped. His head was supported by an anesthetist, who operated a gas machine with his other hand. Three Vietnamese nurses in masks scurried around the room, carrying instruments and drapes.

We continued our tour. Behind surgery was "Trai 12," or Ward 12, a recently completed postoperative area. It housed at least 25 patients—two patients occupied many of the beds. None had mattresses. The springs were covered by reed mats or newspapers. Don said the mattresses had either rotted or been eaten by rats.

Trai 9, another postoperative ward, was surrounded by a pool of stagnant water. Swarms of mosquitoes roiled the turbid waters as we negotiated the obstacle.

"Just call me Andy, sir," Specialist Anderson offered as he applied a forearm cast. The recipient, a small boy, screamed loudly and tried to wrench loose from his captor. Don explained Andy had been working with Doctor Owen in surgery and had experience in medical and pediatric care as well.

A petite Vietnamese girl approached wearing a lovely *áo dài*. Don introduced me to Co Anh, chief nurse of Trai 9. "I am happy to acquaint you," she said with a curtsy, "but you are so young to be a Bac Si!"

The hospital kitchen was our next stop. Inside the smoke-blackened room, three open fires were tended by ageless women—I was reminded of the witches' scene in *Macbeth*. The fires were the product of rice hulls, several bags of which were stacked in one corner. Atop metal supports were iron cauldrons containing soup. In another corner demijohns held rainwater; a pig's carcass hung from a rafter. Near the open doorway two women squatted as they peeled vegetables.

On the hospital grounds I met Sgt. Hale and Spc. Hill, recent team arrivals. Don was called away, so I continued my visit without a guide.

Trai 8, a male medicine ward, was separated from the rest of the hospital by a coconut grove. The walls and floors were brown with dirt. The patients peered at me with curiosity. Like the other wards, beds usually contained two patients as family members squatted nearby. There was no electricity or running water and no hospital personnel in attendance. Adjacent to the ER was Maternity.

Ward 6, the female medicine ward, was cleaner than its male counterpart, although no less crowded and without staff. Opposite Ward 6 was a small structure occupied by ARVN medical personnel. Barbed wire and mud bunkers separated the building from the civilian hospital. The ARVN building was abutted by Ward 3, a government employee ward. On the far side a crumbling structure housed elderly residents. The stench was overpowering.

Behind the kitchen were quarters for hospital personnel, a well, a fishpond, the morgue, and an open field leading to a canal. In front of the kitchen were the nuns' quarters. Pediatrics, or Ward 4, was separated from most of the other buildings, although it featured a cement walk. Linda met me at the front door and hurried me through a hall crowded with patients to the nurses' station.

"Steve usually runs afternoon clinic, but he's on an operation. So, I am the Bac Si today." She twirled a stethoscope in her hand.

"Who is Steve?" I asked.

"He's the MACV doctor but spends most of his spare time here. You'll like him—he's a neat guy."

Two women carrying infants tried to push into the nurses' station but were intercepted by a Vietnamese nurse who ushered them out and closed the door.

"How many patients are out there?" I asked.

"Oh, not many—maybe 30 or so—that's about average for an afternoon clinic." Linda offered.

"Well," I said, "I might as well get my feet wet. If you'll lend me that stethoscope, let's see some patients."

"I hoped you'd say that." she smiled, signaling the nurse to open the door for the first mother and child.

Linda served as my interpreter. There was a seemingly unending procession of sick children. For many I had no clue of the diagnosis. Linda provided helpful advice, including how to write prescriptions for the pharmacy. We admitted a few but most of the kids went home.

"That's the last one," Linda said after the hallway had finally emptied. "Let's make quick rounds before we call it a day."

The pediatric ward contained at least 40 patients, including many infants. We stopped at the bed of one tot who was coughing red frothy sputum, which the mother wiped from the baby's mouth with a dirty rag. I listened to his lungs. "Bilateral pneumonia," I said. "Can we get an IV and some oxygen for this kid?"

"We don't have any oxygen," admitted Linda casually, "and if we start an IV, nobody'll be around to look after it. The nurses go home in a few minutes."

"No nurses at night?" I exclaimed.

"Only on Ward 12 and the ER," Linda said matter-of-factly.

I shook my head in disbelief. "Well, let's give it some fluid by clysis [a needle in the skin with fluid infused into the tissues]—and a shot of penicillin."

That evening I learned hooch life had its drawbacks. My bed was comfortable, but spiders and mosquitoes crawled through holes in the mosquito netting to investigate their new source of food, and a small rat had taken up residence in one corner of the hooch. "Don't mind him," Don admonished as he rose in the morning. "There are lots more where he came from. That's why they call us the paddy rats."

After breakfast Don walked me to the hospital and the MILPHAP office, a converted storeroom.

A thin Vietnamese girl of 20 or so in a white *áo dài* entered the office with a young man in a brown felt hat. Don acknowledged them. "Dick, these are two of our interpreters. Co Phung is our chief interpreter; Mr. Ky works in pediatrics."

"I'm happy to meet you," said Co Phung in perfect English.

"How do you do, Doctor," Mr. Ky offered stiffly, who told me Steve would not cover pediatrics today.

"I guess we'd better get over there," I said as Ky and I headed for the door.

A collection of mothers and infants squatted beside the entrance to pediatrics. An elderly woman with a mop opened the door for us. Linda was at the nurses' station, preparing an injection, along with a pregnant Vietnamese nurse who suppressed a sob as she acknowledged me.

Linda put down the syringe," "That's Ba Hoi," she said. "She always cries when a patient dies."

"Who died?" I asked.

"Two—the kid we saw with pneumonia and another in the third room. Shall we make rounds before clinic?"

We saw 46 patients. It was a blur—I reviewed Owen's notes and those of Steve Reynard. We sent a few kids home and I made chart entries. There was a bewildering variety of illnesses—pneumonia, parasites, common colds, earaches, diarrhea, rashes, and tuberculosis (TB). Many were puzzles, with no specific diagnoses. After rounds I limped through clinic with Linda's help, then met Don who oriented me to MILPHAP activities. He reminded me to pack for a trip to Can Tho the following day to meet with regional USAID health officials.

As we were leaving for the airport the next morning, I met Steve Reynard, the tall, affable doctor who had been helping us in addition to his MACV duties.

"I've got a daily sick call for the compound and have to go on military operations, but I'm happy to see patients in the clinic and the hospital," he said, adding humbly, "If that's OK with you."

He studied my face for a moment. "Say, you look familiar—where'd you go to med school?"

"USC," I replied. "Me too," he chimed in. "In fact, I think I was your intern at LA County." Our conversation was cut short as Don called from the jeep.

We flew to Can Tho and proceeded to USAID headquarters to meet Dr. John Marsh, the public health officer who worked in a predecessor of the MILPHAP program in 1964. A quiet, soft-spoken man, he expressed sincere interest in our hospital and apologized that Dr. Douglas, his superior, was not present to greet us.

Don and I listened as John gave us a run-down on Bac Lieu. He was very complimentary of Dr. Vinh, not only as a surgeon, but an administrator. John explained there were Army, Navy and Air Force MILPHAP teams in IV Corps, as well as Spanish, Philippine, Australian, and Iranian units. "The delta probably has more medical talent than anywhere in Vietnam," he offered. "But it creates a lot of headaches. We've got to supply medicines and equipment to all these hospitals, plus deal with unforeseen issues—like 100 bottles of wine a month for the Spanish team and trying to find Iranian-Vietnamese interpreters. That is, until we learned the Iranians all speak English."

The day passed quickly, and Don and I learned of the many obstacles we would face. At the airport, we waited under the wing of an Air America aircraft. The pilot, a tall Gary Cooper type, squatted nearby.

"What kind of plane is this?" I asked, looking at the long cowling and huge exhausts.

"Porter," replied the droll pilot, picking up a rock and tossing it at a nearby bird.

"They're Swiss," he continued, "but we also build 'em in the States—turbine engine—doesn't have much range, but it'll take off and land in a bean patch—great for this kind of country."

Most Air America (AA) pilots were ex-military and hired for two-year contracts. AA was a branch of the State Department but was covertly owned and operated by the Central Intelligence Agency (CIA). AA provided transportation for USAID and other officials as well as clandestine operations. The plots were well paid and they earned it. Since 1961, more than 60 fliers had been shot down, plus unknown numbers lost during AA's secret operations.

The next morning, I wandered into the operating room to hear the following conversation between two middle-aged men in surgical gowns and masks:

"Golf."

"Gof."

"Golf—Bac Si, you have to add the 'L'."

The exchange involved a Vietnamese man wearing horn-rim glasses and Bill Owen as they performed a hernia repair. Bill looked up as I poked my head in the room.

"We have an arrangement," said Owen. "I teach him English pronunciation, and he tutors me on Vietnamese."

Vinh started to close the fascia but stopped to flick away a fly on the instrument tray. He glanced at me over his glasses.

"Bac Si, this is Dr. Carlson, our new MILPHAP chief doctor," Owen announced. Vinh did not respond but completed a line of sutures and waited for Bill to tie the last knot. Owen closed the skin and both surgeons held the patient who was beginning to arouse from anesthesia. Vinh dressed the wound and removed his gloves. Owen struggled with the patient who was now nearly awake. As the anesthetist removed the endotracheal tube from the patient, Vinh took off his mask, revealing a red crease over his cheeks.

He looked over his glasses and asked blandly, "What do you think of Bac Lieu?" His tone seemed friendly enough, but it was clearly a leading question.

"I don't know, the hospital needs a lot of work," I bit my tongue, regretting my frankness. "There are many sick patients," I said, trying to soften my remarks.

Vinh made no comment and was expressionless. He lit a Ruby Queen cigarette and offered one to Bill and me.

The medicine chief was of average size for a Vietnamese male—about 5 feet 7 inches. His face was broad and tanned, topped by black hair combed to one side, his hands lean and strong. Placing his glasses in a breast pocket, he nodded to the anesthetist to move the patient to a stretcher. Vinh's shirt was a wash-and-wear synthetic fabric of light green color. The top two buttons were open. His grey slacks were also a synthetic material. He wore sandals and no socks. I could not fathom his impression of me.

He turned to me, "You are the only doctor for the team—the last one had three doctors."

"We should be getting more," I offered meekly.

Vinh sighed visibly, "I hope you like Bac Lieu."

He limply shook my hand, patted Owen on the shoulder, and walked out.

"I don't think I made a very good impression," I said.

Bill handed the patient's chart to a nurse, who directed two women to remove the patient from the operating room. "Oh, I wouldn't worry about it. Vinh takes a while to know—inscrutable Oriental and all that, you know."

That evening a knock on our hooch door interrupted me as I typed the day's events. A tall, thin captain wearing tropical fatigues entered. "Am I bothering you?" he asked. "I'm Stoney Burton—we've not met."

"Dick Carlson—glad to meet you." We shook hands and Stoney took a chair.

"I work with Steve. Don said you will be our new MOC."

"I suppose—although I don't have much to command now. But I hear more folks are coming."

"Well, if I can help you out—you know, supplies and things like that. Let me know. Sometimes I can get stuff that isn't available through regular channels."

He pointed to the typewriter. "Looks like we have another 'gray ghost.'" "Who's that?" I asked.

"Colonel Maddox—our commander. That's his call sign. He types reports almost every night. What're you writing—a book?"

"Just a journal—I've never done one before—I thought it'd be a way to recall my experiences and pass the time."

He rose and paused as he opened the door. "Be sure to spell my name right."

Stoney wore an army uniform, but his routine differed from other officers and he rarely participated in military operations with the ARVN division. It was suspected he had other duties—such as with the CIA. He came to our rescue on several occasions, arranging flights by Air America and miraculously securing needed supplies.

My daily typed entry became a compulsion as I recorded events and conversations as accurately as possible. Despite fatigue and competition from other tasks, I strived to be objective, but emotion and opinion filtered into my comments. I also typed letters to my family and friends, such as instructions for where to purchase 16 mm movie film at a Hollywood photo shop and requests for personal items. This was before packages were subject to X-ray or other probes. Virtually anything could be shipped. Some individuals even transported weapons via the mail, which was very efficient. Food, gifts, clothes, even bottles of wine, would arrive within days.

During my initial days in Bac Lieu, I observed no wartime activity by the VC or the ARVN division, which was headquartered adjacent to the compound, although my military education began at breakfast.

Two captains were discussing an intelligence report. An ARVN outpost had been overrun just before dawn. Five soldiers were killed plus multiple injured, including dependents who lived with the soldiers. The VC moved swiftly and were gone before helicopter and ground support could arrive.

"How often does something like that happen?" I asked.

"Nearly every night if you consider the DTA," explained one of the officers.

"The DTA," he continued, "is the Division Tactical Area and includes several delta provinces. It is the operational area for the 21st ARVN division—the soldiers we advise and support. It's a huge region."

"Do they ever hit a big town like Bac Lieu?"

"Occasionally. The last time was 1965. They could attack us anytime, although I doubt if they will," he laughed. "Too many of 'em live here. Besides, our 105s keep them off guard at night." He reminded me that most nights we would be serenaded by the 105 mm ARVN howitzers located adjacent to the compound, which fired H&I (Harassment & Interdiction) rounds at suspected enemy positions.

Moments later Col. Maddox entered the mess hall. There was a momentary pause as everyone observed the presence of the commanding officer. The colonel sat with his executive officer at a table designated "SA and Staff." Maddox was a strikingly handsome man of above average height; lean and muscular, with a shock of silver hair, origin of the moniker "grey ghost." He could have just stepped off a Hollywood set and reminded me of Rock Hudson or Gregory Peck.

Saturday's clinic was light, perhaps 15 to 18 kids. The hospital was officially closed except for emergencies. After clinic I walked the grounds and made a crude map of the establishment.

Most vacant land was occupied by puddles and coconut palms and there was ample room for expansion. I thought new construction as well as renovation of existing structures would be worthy goals for our team. None of the structures except the operating suite had glass windows. Only maternity and Ward 12 had screens, and

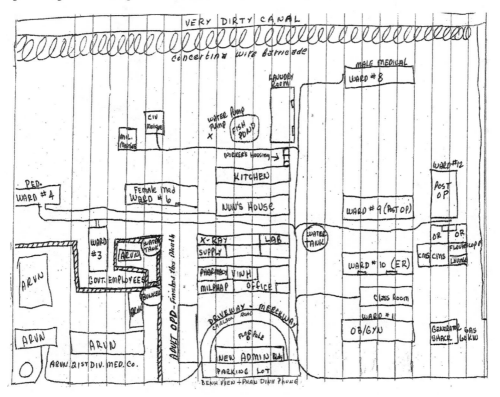

My drawing/map of hospital.

the only indoor flush toilet was in the surgical suite, which was inoperative and mal-odorous. Patients, relatives, animals, and townspeople ate, cooked, and defecated throughout the hospital grounds, compounding sanitary problems. Used dressings, bandages, and other trash were carried to a dump behind Ward 8, where children and dogs picked through the debris before burning. The morgue was a small build-ing with peeling paint and a cement and sheet metal autopsy table in the center of the dank room. "This is not a morgue," I said aloud to myself, "it's an abattoir."

The rear of the administration building housed the small X-ray machine and laboratory. A smiling young technician showed me her meager facility as she said the lab could process simple blood counts, smears for TB or other bacteria, blood crossmatching for transfusion, urinalysis, and exam of stool for parasites. Cultures were sent to Can Tho and required several days. Routine laboratory studies in the United States such as serum electrolytes and others that required electronic analyz-ers were not available. I thought, "Clinical judgment will be our guide—I hope I'm up to the task."

I made evening rounds with Bill Owen; his flashlight furnished illumination for our journey through the darkened wards. We picked our way to Ward 4 as bats dipped around us. Several families anticipated his arrival and greeted him with open palms. "Xin Bac Si—thouc dau," they intoned.

"They want pain, or 'dau' medicine," Bill said, remov-ing a bottle from his pocket to shake out several aspirin pills to extended hands.

We made our way through the wards and Bill listened to a few patients' lungs and per-formed brief physical exams. "We can't do much," admitted Owen, "but if someone is really sick, we can send them to the ER or Ward 12."

Returning to the compound, two rats trotted across our path. "They look healthier than most of the patients," I observed.

Sunday was crisp and cooler. I made rounds on Pediatrics and walked to Ward 12 with Steve. Bill was examining a young girl's leg. "Take a look at this," he said. Below the girl's knee was a gigantic open defect exposing the bone. The wound was badly

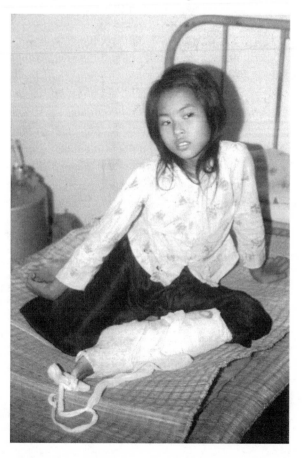

Child with leg infection that required amputation.

infected. The girl winced as the nurse poured disinfectant over the wound. She was a beautiful child, probably eight years of age.

Steve and I shook our heads and uttered in unison, "Osteo [osteomyelitis— infection of the bone]."

Bill nodded agreement. "I'm not sure we can save this leg, but we'll pump her full of antibiotics and debride. I'll show her to Dr. Vinh tomorrow. As long as you are here, I should let you see the rest of the horror show."

He led us to the next room as relatives scurried from our path. We stopped at a child's bed. The right side of her face was covered with bandages.

Bill told the story. "Grenade—she lost an eye, and her parents were killed by the blast. She cried for nearly two weeks, but now we've got her to smile a little."

Outside we saw Co Anh sitting on the stoop, clad in a light-colored *áo dài*. She was reading a book entitled *Intermediate English*. "Chao Bac Si," she offered as she rose.

"Chao Co," responded Bill. "Where is the Cambodian boy?"

She led us to a corner of the ward. The boy, probably 16 years or so, was lying face down on a cot. Both legs had been amputated at the thigh. He smiled as we approached, exposing three gold teeth.

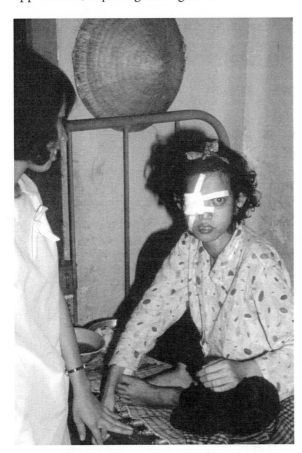

Girl with traumatic loss of eye.

"This fellow was a VC about a year ago," explained Bill. "He was shot in the back during a raid. The VC left him to die, but an ARVN brought him here. He's been a paraplegic ever since."

"But why the amputations?" asked Steve.

"The rats started eating his toes, so ..."

"What?" I exclaimed.

"Oh, he couldn't feel it of course, but it's enough to give you the creeps. The wards are crawling with them at night. Owen handed the boy a cigarette, who laughed as he puffed, playfully blowing smoke at us.

"Anyway," continued Owen, "they were forced to keep revising the amputations higher and higher as rats ate through his dressings. Now there is nothing left of his legs."

Co Anh tugged at Bill's sleeve, "Isn't it time to go, Bac Si?"

"Where are you going?" asked Steve.

"Church—Co Phung is coming too," Bill offered.

"But aren't they Buddhist?" I looked at Co Anh—"Aren't you Buddhist?" I stammered.

Bill answered, "Yes, but they like to go—and it helps their English."

He turned to Co Anh and offered a compliment of her *áo dài*: "Dep Lam [beautiful]."

The *áo dài* has been the traditional garb for Vietnamese for nearly 200 years. The female version is the most common and includes a tight-fitting tunic with free-floating back and front flaps which cover flowing trousers. The entire gown is silk and pastel or white, which may contrast the tunic and trousers. The fabric is thin, although men wear a version with thicker material.

"It is the national dress of Vietnam," she explained, blushing somewhat. Turning to me she asked, "Would you like to learn Vietnamese?"

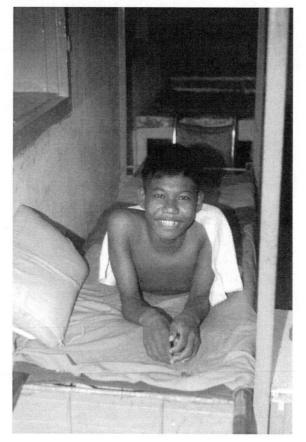

Paraplegic Cambodian boy with thigh amputations from rats eating his wounds.

I nodded yes.

"I will teach you. Tomorrow we go downtown to buy a book."

The next morning Pat was having an argument on Trai 8, the male medicine ward, as we arrived. She turned to Bill for assistance. "They won't let me take temperatures. He says it ruins his charts." She pointed to the male nurse, a young man looking somewhat guilty, wearing a dirty smock, brown trousers, and sandals. Pat continued, "I don't know why we keep records anyway; Bac Si Koung never looks at 'em."

"Khoung," Bill explained, "is the Vietnamese doctor in charge of this ward. I don't come here unless Pat asks for help. Khoung is not our best physician."

Bill glanced at an empty bed. "Did he die?"

"The man in the next bed said his relatives took him away before dawn. He wasn't sure if the man had already died." Her voice trailed off. "That's our second tetanus death in three days."

"Well, at least you made them get rid of the snakes," Bill said in an effort to cheer her.

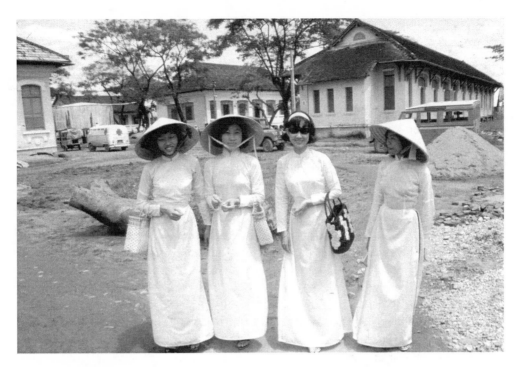

Interpreters and secretary in *áo dàis*: Co Tuyet, Co Trien, Co Phung, and Co Ha (secretary).

He looked at me. "Several patients kept pet snakes—it drove Pat nuts until she finally was able to have them removed."

I learned more of Dr. Khoung as we walked to Ward 9. He was an older physician and would retire soon or go to the military. He was not precise in his diagnoses or treatments. Like many of the local Bac Si's, he liberally used cortisone, strychnine, and camphor. Camphor was given as an injection, which is very painful, making the medicine more powerful according to locals. "'A pain for a pain,' is the motto," Bill explained, adding Khoung was known to give TB patients cortisone, but no anti–TB medications. In the States that would be gross malpractice. Khoung had resisted all offers to help run his ward, and Pat was constantly frustrated by the poor medical care. Bill suggested if Khoung changed his practices because of the Americans, he would "lose face," diminishing his authority and humiliating him. He also spent more time in his downtown private practice than at the hospital—a typical scenario of many VN doctors who worked in province hospitals.

"We have to be patient and make progress where we can," Bill offered philosophically.

After lunch I drove Co Anh downtown. At a small sidewalk shop she selected a book of Vietnamese-to-English translation. The book's cover featured the drawing of a boy and girl. She took out a pencil and wrote, "Bac Si Carlson" and "Co Anh" under the pictures.

A technician from Can Tho brought a new X-ray tube in the afternoon. I was elated until Don showed me the wiring in the back of the larger machine. "Those wires aren't enough to handle a Christmas tree, let alone an X-ray machine," he said, pointing to the mess. "If we hook it up, it'll just blow the tube again, or cause a fire. We need to rewire the whole hospital." We thanked the technician, carefully wrapped the tube, and stored it in our hooch.

Sick babies occupied my evening. One infant was severely dehydrated from diarrhea. Each breath appeared to be its last. We started an IV and instructed its parents to remove the needle when the fluid was exhausted. The baby's chances were poor, and he died later that night.

Steve and I paused on the steps of Ward 9 after rounds, enjoying the night air. The sky was clear, and the shadows masked the daytime ugliness of the hospital. Behind us palm trees whispered in response to the ocean breezes, producing a sound similar to running water.

Suddenly our reverie was interrupted by the sound of the hospital generator and a blaze of light from the surgery center. We beheld Dr. Vinh clad in pajamas, sitting on a bench outside the surgery center, smoking a cigar. Two patients lay on stretchers in the hallway. One had a gunshot wound, the other a woman with an ectopic pregnancy. Steve and I watched as Owen assisted Vinh, who had impressive surgical skill—fast, decisive, and adept. He quickly isolated bleeding vessels and secured hemostasis. As both patients were in shock, the procedures required rapid action. Steve remarked of Vinh, "He must have ice-water in his veins." Owen nodded, reminding us it's necessary under the circumstances.

A normal pregnancy occurs after an ovum is released approximately mid-menstrual cycle, travels to the fallopian tube, and is fertilized by a sperm. The zygote migrates to the uterus and is implanted, and the embryo grows to become a fetus. An ectopic pregnancy occurs when the fertilized egg remains outside the uterus. Causes include a sexually transmitted disease, endometriosis, or ovarian abnormalities. Pain and life-threatening bleeding result, with significant maternal mortality. Ectopics were frequent causes of emergency surgery in Bac Lieu, although we never learned why.

After morning rounds, I was directed to the morgue where Vinh was performing an autopsy. A young ARVN had hung himself a few days earlier. Family and curious onlookers, including many giggling children, crowded the area. The smell was nauseating. A cigarette dangling from his mouth, Vinh calmly dissected the body, expressionless as usual. He was not only the provincial chief health officer—but also coroner. I shook my head as I returned to the ward.

Later we examined the girl with osteomyelitis. Her leg remained badly infected. Antibiotics and local treatments had yielded little effect. I asked Bill, "Has Vinh seen her yet?"

"Yeah—he took one look and went, 'psst.' The leg may have to come off, but I don't want to be the one to do it."

The girl looked at us inquisitively—she cocked her head to one side and regarded us with amusement but not fear.

Bill changed topics. "Vinh is operating on a boy with an eye wound this afternoon. Do you want to watch?"

"Sure," I said. "Where did Vinh learn plastic surgery? He certainly is a man of many talents."

Bill remarked, "He went to medical school in Hanoi—graduated in the '40s. He spent a few years in the army and picked up some surgical techniques from the French. I think he was involved in fighting between the Viet Minh and the French. He may have gone to France briefly."

"Some of his techniques seem a bit old fashioned," I suggested.

Owen shot back, "Don't underestimate him—what he lacks in polish he makes up with guts and experience."

"I didn't mean he was …" I had obviously touched a tender chord.

"Do you know," Bill continued in a softer tone, "Vinh is the only surgeon for nearly 300,000 people? He's seen more injuries than most trauma surgeons in the States—to say nothing of the routine stuff. They told me he was offered a professor post in Saigon but turned it down to stay in the sticks. That's guts—and dedication. He's probably one of the best medicine chiefs in the country—if not the best."

That afternoon I watched as Vinh and Bill operated on the boy with the eye wound. Vinh's glasses were low on his nose, and he was quietly but swiftly performing a skin flap. It was clear he had done many such procedures. There was little conversation. The only sound was the boy breathing through the gas machine as the anesthetist squeezed the rubber bag.

When finished, we adjourned to the dressing room where three "ba moi ba'" beers had thoughtfully been placed on the desk. Vinh removed his glasses and took a long drink.

"Perhaps you should have helped," he said, looking at me, "my eyes are more tired each year."

I placed my beer on the desk, popped out a contact lens and placed it in his hand, "My eyes are already tired." He didn't recognize it immediately, but then smiled and we all had a good laugh.

The following day was Thanksgiving. MACV took a holiday from the war but patients hadn't been told of the American institution. Clinics held their usual capacity. I admitted a boy with scrofula (TB of the neck). Neither Steve nor I had ever seen a case except in textbooks. The obliging young man posed as we photographed his lesions.

Lunch, actually Thanksgiving dinner, was a treat. The mess hall featured pictures of turkeys, pilgrims, and Indians, and the meal had all the trimmings. Vinh accepted our invitation and was amused by the decorations.

My meal was interrupted by the telephone. As there was no direct communication between the hospital and our quarters, the prior team improvised a message system. Mimeographed sheets printed in VN and English were kept in the ER. To call a doctor, the nurse checked the symptom or condition, carried the note to the rear gate where the guard telephoned our hooch, officers club, or mess hall. Today's note simply read: Wounds.

Co Anh was waiting for me at the gate. "Please hurry, Bac Si—very bad."

The boy was cradled in his mother's arms. He had been shot through the left flank, the bullet coursing through the abdomen and exiting beside the right nipple. He was dead.

I looked at Co Anh and a student worker standing next to the mother. To my amazement the worker smiled and managed a suppressed giggle. Co Anh glared at the girl, then told the family the boy was dead and to take him away. The family began wailing and sobbing, pulling their hair and pounding the floor. But they heeded Co Anh's words and soon the parents and the dead child were on a cyclo, heading into the unknown.

Steve was the hero of evening rounds. He hit one of the rats outside Ward 4 with a rock. "Be careful," joked Bill, as the rodent limped off, "he's going for reinforcements."

A celebrity arrived on the morning Caribou—a reporter from *Time* magazine. His writing may have been lucid, but his appearance resembled Hollywood casting—slouch hat, beard, camouflaged fatigues, and a Leica around his neck. He came to document a divisional operation for an article on MACV and ARVN units, but remained aloof and didn't engage any of the MACV officers at dinner.

The operation was postponed, and men spent the day playing cards, taping music, or sunbathing. Our literary visitor remained in the air-conditioned officers' club.

Joan Schubert, the chief USAID nurse, returned from R&R and I met her in the MILPHAP office. She was a light-haired woman of medium height, perhaps 30 years of age, who was outgoing but all business. I found her approach refreshing, but she and Don had not hit it off.

My introduction to the war began as a bus brought casualties from the village of Gia Rai. A girl of 12 stepped on a claymore mine. Three other patients suffered minor wounds. Bill came to help with the girl's amputation. It is not a pleasant task to cut off a young person's leg. An ARVN operation was held the next morning.

The "thud-thud" of choppers merged with the drone of conventional aircraft, disturbing the predawn solitude. I had just returned from the hospital ER when alarm clocks in adjacent hooches rang. It was 4:30 a.m., and the compound roused in preparation for war. Soon my neighbors had dressed and departed, and the compound was again quiet. The officers did not return until 5:00 p.m. I asked a tired Tom Needham how it had gone.

"Nothing to it—a walk in the paddies," he replied easily. "Eight VC killed, 2 ARVN—about average for a small operation." He removed his sweaty clothes and joined others in the showers.

My Vietnamese lessons began that evening. Co Anh and I sat on the steps of Ward 9 until the light faded. She started with simple phrases, days of the week, numbers, and greetings. The language is not grammatically difficult but is tonal. The seven tones, combined with the monosyllabic characteristic of the language, create many words with similar construction, but many meanings. However, one positive outcome of the French colonial era was to convert the language's Chinese characters to a Latin alphabet.

A pair of writer-photographers from *Life* magazine met Bill and me at lunch. They were writing an article on AMA volunteer physicians and planned to use Bill Owen as their lead. Sam Angelof and Dick Swanson soon learned their potential subject was less than enthusiastic.

"Can't you use someone else?" Bill asked, "Isn't there another doctor you can write about. There's lots of men over here far more interesting than me."

"But don't you want to put…, where'd you say you were from in Iowa?" asked Dick.

"St. Ansgar," responded Bill.

"Yeah, St. Ansgar—don't you want to put St. Ansgar on the map?"

"Not particularly," Owen affirmed, buttering a roll. "I'm just doing a job—there's nothing very special about that."

Sam moved a chair closer to Bill and began taking notes on a yellow tablet as Dick pressed his reluctant subject, "Well, the folks in Saigon recommended you as the typical Project Vietnam doctor. We think you'll make a good subject." Warming to his topic, he continued, "You know, a lot of doctors in the States will see this, and maybe it'll get more volunteers."

Owen was weakening, "Just what do you want me to do?"

Dick sensed victory. "Nothing—just your daily routine. We'll follow you around and try to stay out of the way."

Owen reluctantly agreed, and the two newsmen spent the afternoon asking questions and taking photos of Bill. On evening rounds Dick shot more film as Sam took notes. Dick had two Nikons and a tripod for time exposures by candlelight or flashlight. The patients paid little attention to the guests.

The following morning Bill and Vinh performed several surgeries as Dick shot pictures. Vinh expressed interest in Dick's equipment and after one operation asked to examine Dick's Nikon, then trotted to his office, returning with a Leica.

Dick was amused, "I think he works for *NEWSWEEK*," he laughed.

Vinh insisted Dick and Sam pose with Owen as he snapped pictures with his Leica.

Later, we learned another MILPHAP doctor would join our team within a few days, a fully trained obstetrician.

My first month passed with occasional episodes of violence by VC or ARVN, but no attacks had occurred in Bac Lieu, a situation which would soon change—the delta war was heating up.

Chapter Sources

Jack Langguth. "A New GI Argot Can Be Heard in Vietnam: Hooches (Barracks)." *New York Times*, September 20, 1964.

G. B. Chamberlain. "Honcho, Hooch, and Hooch Honcho." *American Speech* 60, no. 4 (1985): 370–72.

Richard W. Carlson. *Bac Si My: Volunteer Physicians for Vietnam* [Film]. American Medical Association, 1968.

Dushman, Amber. "AMA Volunteer Physicians for Vietnam." Personal communication, March 8, 2019.

Kelsey Walsh. "Volunteer Service From American Physicians During the Vietnam War." *AMA Journal of Ethics* 21, no. 9 (2019): E806–12.

Gabriel Smilkstein. "Volunteer Physicians for Vietnam." *JAMA* 219, no. 4 (1972): 495–9.

"The 'Bac Si' from Iowa." *Life Magazine*, February 17, 1967, 78a–82.

Kurt T. Barnhart. "Ectopic Pregnancy." *New England Journal of Medicine* 361, no. 4 (2009): 379–87.

5

December

Bombs, Gifts, and Baby Soup

I was examining an infant in the clinic when I received a note. "Vinh is starting surgery and wants you to scrub. Hurry!"

The procedure was in progress when I arrived, another ectopic pregnancy. I quickly scrubbed, gowned, and stepped across the operating table from Vinh, who was struggling with several bleeding sites. As he clamped the fallopian tube, he smiled at me through his mask. He rapidly controlled the blood loss, but the anesthetist leaned over and whispered in his ear.

"Blood pressure is low," Vinh translated. He stepped back and asked me to close the abdomen. I told the anesthetist to give some dextran to raise the blood pressure. When I looked up, Vinh had gone. As I sutured the fascia, I realized Vinh was allowing me to flex my surgical skills and assume more responsibility. I thought, "He isn't testing me—he's encouraging me."

Our care of sick infants and children was complicated by severe malnutrition, unfortunately worsened by the Vietnamese nurses. One morning I observed Ba Hoi, the pediatric head nurse, preparing formula for her charges. She was adding powdered milk to a pan of water atop a small gas stove. Her staff would give each child a portion of the mixture. Fresh or reconstituted cow's milk was a rarity in Bac Lieu, which had no commercial dairies, and canned or powdered milk was very expensive. Accordingly, Vietnamese mothers nursed three or more years. Cultural issues played a role, as powdered milk was not accepted by many peasants. I winced as I watched as the Ba added a few spoonfuls of powdered milk to two cups of water—a very dilute result with little nutritional benefit.

Steve spent the evening at the MACV aid station, removing plexiglass shards from the pilot of an L-19 "shotgun," or forward air control plane (FAC). The windshield of the tiny craft had been hit by a sniper's bullet—spraying the pilot's chest and face with multiple fragments.

The following day, Co Anh joined Owen, Don, and me and several pediatric patients for a trip to a Chinese restaurant downtown. Dick Swanson accompanied us as we loaded the paraplegic Cambodian boy and other kids into the USAID Scout. The restaurant's owner directed us to a table, and we enjoyed soup, shrimp, crab, fish, and a variety of vegetables. The lunch was a huge success as the young patients giggled throughout the meal to the delight of the photographer.

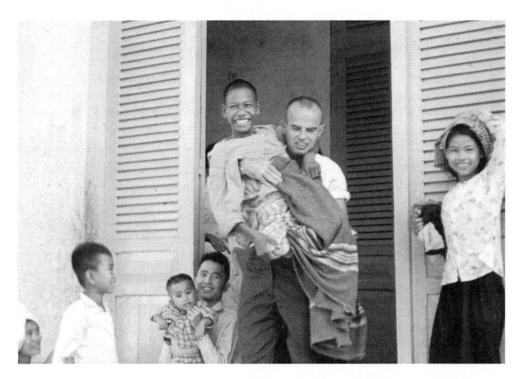

Hospital kids, Dr. Owen carrying paraplegic Cambodian boy to lunch downtown.

The arrival of the morning 'bou was delayed. Tan Son Nuht airport had been shelled with considerable damage and several American fatalities. The MACV headquarters where I had been quartered was also attacked. War seemed to be getting closer.

Clinics were closed, so I walked downtown to obtain a better picture of Bac Lieu. I was immediately surrounded by a group of curious children shouting, "Chao Bac Si." They were eager for handouts, so I bought 10 piastres of candy. After satisfying themselves no additional gifts were forthcoming, the kids abandoned me.

The town was bisected by a main canal and featured two or three dirt streets lined with small shops and open-air restaurants. There was no array of sidewalk black-market vendors as in Saigon, and the shops were neat. Although it was Sunday, stores were open and busy, including a market with fruits, vegetables, and a variety of fish, crabs, and shrimp. Other shops sold dry goods, pots, pans, and various cooking devices.

Dr. Owen led evening rounds, replete with flashlights, stethoscopes, and Dick Swanson's Nikon. When I returned to our hooch, Don reminded me we would fly to Saigon in the morning to USAID headquarters to see Col. Moncrief.

We motored to the airport where an Air America Beechcraft was on the tarmac. We were the only passengers, and I sat in the copilot's seat. Nearing Saigon, the pilot pointed to several UH-l "Huey" gunships making runs over a tree-lined canal, dropping ordnance, firing machine guns and rockets. The spectacle was akin to a World War II movie. Hueys that carried troops were termed "slicks." Heavier armed choppers with rockets, grenade launchers, M-60 machine guns, or 20 mm cannons were called "hogs."

We met Col. Moncrief, who updated us on the magnitude of public health problems in Bac Lieu and our role—a daunting task, even in peacetime. He acknowledged the difficulties but was optimistic, and cited contributions of PHAP teams. He said we were lucky to work with Dr. Vinh and was very complimentary of the medicine chief. Following the Colonel's comments, we proceeded to Phu Tho, a gigantic warehouse that housed thousands of hospital items—autoclaves, operating tables, lamps, X-ray machines, everything needed to outfit a modern facility. We collected items on our list and returned to our billet.

Rising early, we loaded our goods in a cab and drove to Tan Son Nhut to join the world's largest air traffic jam. We arrived in time for the evening call.

At 3:00 a.m., I was awakened to see a child with fever and convulsions. My flashlight was not working, and the mother held a candle as I examined the boy. He was in terrible condition; I wrote some orders for seizure medications, cooling, and antibiotics. He probably had meningitis. I returned to my hooch, but couldn't sleep, knowing the child would have a better chance in a modern facility.

Dr. Owen and Vinh operated on a boy with a cleft lip and palate. Congenital lesions were common in Vietnam but infrequently repaired because of lack of surgical care. Vinh was the only surgeon within 100 miles with plastic surgery training. After surgery Bill sat on a bed, exhausted after another long day treating Bac Lieu's inhabitants.

On their final night in Bac Lieu, the *LIFE* correspondents dutifully trudged through the mud and darkness for evening rounds. The main attraction was the rats on Pediatrics. In the dim light, Dick Swanson shot several photos of doctors tossing stones at the rodents.

Later, Owen and I were called to the ER for a woman with cholera. She was very dehydrated with low blood pressure. We inserted two IVs to help restore her blood pressure and gave fluid rapidly. To our delight, within an hour she was alert and talking to her family as we left.

Cholera is an intestinal infection from fecal-contaminated food or water with the bacteria *Vibrio cholera*. The result is profuse diarrhea. In Vietnam, outbreaks are seasonal due to changes in water salinity and temperature. Untreated fatality may exceed 50 percent. Profuse diarrhea,

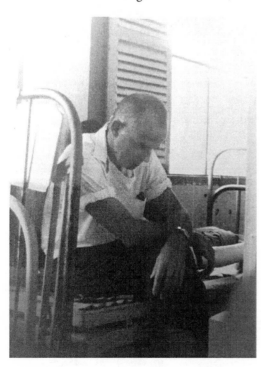

An exhausted Dr. Owen on a hospital bed.

termed "rice water stools," leads to severe dehydration and shock. Although an infection, cholera does not cause fever or other signs of inflammation. In the mid–1800s, John Snow, Queen Victoria's physician, was the first to identify contaminated water as the source of transmission, dispelling centuries of myths of the disease's origin.

The mechanism leading to diarrhea is unique. The bacteria elaborate an enterotoxin, which alters the ability of intestinal cells to produce the chemical adenyl cyclase, inhibiting reabsorption of intestinal juice. The result is profound diarrhea. If the loss of diarrheal fluid can be offset by oral or IV fluids, the defect is reversible. Antibiotics hasten recovery, but the mainstay of therapy is vigorous fluid resuscitation. In the late 1800s Robert Koch identified the organism and observed recovery provided immunity, paving the way for a vaccine. There were no reports of Americans infected with cholera in VN.

The pediatric ward was bursting at the seams—all beds were occupied, some by two or three patients. I admitted four kids from the clinic. Ba Hoi was not pleased, but gracefully accepted her new charges. She was a devoted and sympathetic individual whose gentle tears bespoke concern for patients. She had three children and was seven months pregnant. Although overtaxed, she always had a pleasant disposition and friendly smile. Bill enjoyed working with the kids and had a knack to get them to cooperate. Bill Owen and I were called from lunch to the ER. When we arrived, we beheld a dead child. I also learned the boy I admitted with meningitis had expired. I began afternoon clinic, depressed and frustrated.

The 'bou delivered a huge amount of mail. Friends and relatives sent holiday candy, toys, and other treats for hospital children. Our hooch looked like a dime store at Christmas.

Bac Si Tot oversaw the female medicine ward and invited us to accompany her on rounds. She had not previously allowed American doctors in the female ward or maternity, and we

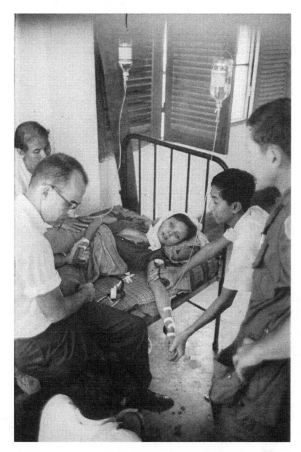

Patient's father, Dr. Owen, cholera patient, Vietnamese nurse, and author as we gave vigorous IV therapy (Dick Swanson/The LIFE Images Collection/Getty Images).

viewed this opening as a rare opportunity for collegiality. The tour was enlighten-ing, and we gained respect for her medical judgment. We saw leprosy, TB, hepati-tis, parasites, and a variety of other medical problems, all managed professionally. After rounds she asked if I would be interested in the maternity service. Dr. Tot was called for difficult deliveries and gynecological issues. The midwives had no experi-ence with forceps. If an infant could not be delivered, the midwives employed a fetal destruction kit, a ghastly set of instruments rarely used in the States. I could not help a furtive glance at Dr. Tot, who was seven months pregnant.

Dinner was interrupted by a hospital call. The message read, "Vet Thuong [war wound]." A three-year-old girl had been shot two days ago and arrived by sampan. Her wound was superficial, involving the right axilla, but badly infected. She was from a VC-controlled area. We asked no questions of her parents' allegiance; they calmly held the crying child as we cleaned and dressed the area.

That evening I practiced my Vietnamese with Co Anh, who corrected my errors and increased my vocabulary, including the term for coconut—"trai dua." The coco-nut served many functions in Vietnam and it was rumored VC medics used coconut milk in lieu of IV fluids.

On Sunday, Don and Bill Owen accompanied the chaplain on his flight around the delta to conduct services at smaller outposts, leaving Steve and me as hospital co-chiefs.

It didn't take long to utilize our services. At noon the ER called us for a patient from Gia Rai with a "may bay" (airplane) injury. The man was unconscious from a head wound. We tried to control the bleeding, but he suddenly had a convulsion and died despite our efforts. Although the nurses told us he was a VC, I completed the application for government compensation for his widow.

A few hours later I was called to maternity for a postpartum woman with bleed-ing. The cause was an undelivered twin. The cervix was contracted, preventing deliv-ery of the second dead child. I called Pat who administered ether to put the mother to sleep and relax the uterus, allowing me to extract the dead child. The next hour included a desperate search for oxytoxic medication to contract the uterus and stem the bleeding. The husband donated blood, and after three hectic hours, we stabilized the mother. I silently thanked my OB instructors at LA County and Pat's help.

The evening brought an unpleasant interchange with a MACV captain. As we tended our steaks on the barbecue, he asked about my day. I told him of the man with the head wound. When he learned of the incident, he became irate. "Those damn VC should all be shot! One minute they are farmers; the next they're shooting at you. We kill a few, but the wounded come crawling to you claiming to be innocent bystanders. Hell, the only way to win a guerrilla war is to kill 'em all!"

I asked how he knew the man was VC, but this further angered him. I secured my steak and retreated to a table, thinking if I were fired upon every day, I'd prob-ably have a similar attitude. But women and children arriving daily with horrific wounds was shocking, and even prisoners of war deserved treatment. I typed that night: "There are no good wars; all lead to more suffering of the innocent than the combatants." My views of the conflict were evolving. The officer's remarks were not typical, but I would encounter others with similar feelings.

Steve left early the next morning for a divisional operation. Injuries that involved U.S. forces were evacuated by "dust off" (medevac) choppers to regional U.S. military hospitals, but Steve remained at the CP (command post) for immediate medical needs. He was near the battles, often at alarmingly close range.

I spent another day in pediatrics, but Bill took night call, allowing me to read. As I sat at the desk, I became fascinated by a small rat that scurried upside down along our hooch's rafters. The rodent was carrying pieces of a white substance in his mouth. Suddenly, I realized he had found our cache of Christmas candy. I awakened Don and we put the goodies in our hot boxes with secure doors.

The next afternoon Steve and MACV officers returned from the two-day operation, tired and dirty, although Steve was in an excited mood. The action occurred at Vi Thang, 50 miles northwest of Bac Lieu. The first day he read a book as he sat on a fuel drum at the airstrip. His only emergency was to treat a helicopter pilot. A bullet entered the starboard door of his craft, shattered the pilot's right arm, and spent itself in the port dash. Following Steve's impromptu surgery, the pilot was evacuated to a field hospital. Steve told me the cockpit was covered with blood and it had been difficult to stem the bleeding.

The second day, Col. Maddox allowed Steve to observe from a thrilling, if not dangerous, perch—a gunship, or hog. Steve's description of rockets, machine guns, and other weapons operated by the chopper's crew was awesome. A battalion-sized unit of VC had been surprised by ARVN forces, and more than 60 of their prisoners were repatriated during the operation. Steve was among the first to reach the prisoners, many of whom were in poor condition. They were evacuated to Can Tho.

I had developed a routine for my daily activities: I skipped breakfast, allowing another 20 minutes of sleep; showered, followed by letter writing and reading. At 8:00 a.m. I made my pilgrimage to the hospital, pockets brimming with VN phrase book, candy, stethoscope, camera, and otoscope. Linda and I would make rounds on Pediatrics, followed by the clinic. At noon I would meet Don to review administrative issues, then wander to surgery to

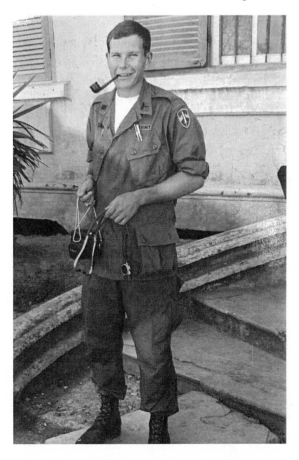

Author, ready for the day outside the hospital.

watch or assist Vinh and Owen complete the morning OR schedule. Lunch was taken at the mess hall, followed by siesta with basketball, tennis, typing, or reading. The hospital reopened at 2:00 p.m., with additional clinical duties. Dinner followed, with hospital call or an evening in the Paddy Rat lounge for drinks or a movie. The day ended typing my journal. Although the clatter of my portable machine may have disturbed my neighbors, I never received a complaint.

Steve had another exciting day in a gunship. Their chopper landed near a group of ARVN troops. Suddenly, multiple explosions rocked the area, sending shrapnel in all directions. Three choppers were damaged, and one American was wounded. Steve was less than 100 yards from the largest explosion of a 250-pound claymore mine buried in the runway. The mine was "command-detonated," meaning the perpetrator was nearby. The blast completely disabled one helicopter and formed a crater 30 feet wide and 10 feet deep. Two other mines exploded but caused less damage. All aircraft that could fly were soon airborne, joined by additional choppers and fixed-wing craft. VC were discovered in surrounding trees, which were transformed into a deadly inferno by rockets, machine guns, and bombs. One man was captured near the strip, still clutching the trip wire to one of the mines.

Steve became my surrogate reporter for the delta war. He participated in divisional operations and had a ring-side seat to the fighting. Officers trusted Steve and took him into their confidence. Although a few exhibited the blind rage and bigotry I experienced at the BBQ, most officers respected the tenacity of the enemy, but not their acts of atrocity. U.S. news agencies reported a progressive increase of the conflict's intensity and rising U.S. antiwar sentiment. But the chain of command and military allegiance were strong—most officers believed the war was justified—while some would not give an opinion or simply wanted to end their tour and go home. MACV officers often developed close bonds with their ARVN colleagues, but racism, mistrust, and confusion undercut the feelings of some advisors, as I was to observe.

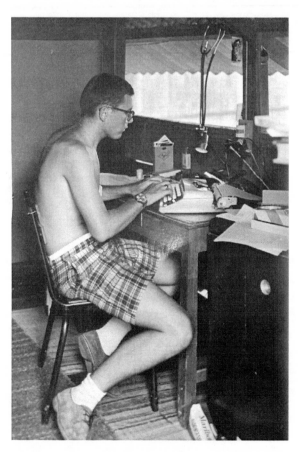

Author, typing my daily journal.

Bill took morning Pediatric duty, allowing me to help with surgical cases. At lunchtime we loaded Owen's car with two patients—the girl whose leg had been amputated and the boy who had lost his parents. Neither child had been out of the hospital for a month. We ate downtown at the same open-air restaurant as before, to the delight of the children and curious onlookers.

Evening call was occupied by gunshot wounds from Gia Rai, the origin of many casualties throughout the year. A total of six were injured in the melee; all but two were children. Vinh was summoned and the surgeries required several hours.

On free afternoons, I struggled with the pronunciation of Vietnamese words with Co Anh's coaching as giggling children observed my vocal attempts. "Trai, phai, mai, and lai" all sounded alike to me, especially with the tonal emphasis.

Bill Owen admitted two Cambodian boys who had been shot by an aircraft near Gia Rai. Their parents were killed in the attack along with several VC. The older boy was struck in the neck, the bullet severing the jugular vein. Fortunately, we ligated the vessel, and the bullet was easily extracted. His younger brother was less fortunate. A machine gun slug traversed his abdomen, damaging multiple organs before finally exiting the left flank. We operated with Vinh and Bill and I donated blood, but the boy expired at 2:00 a.m. The victims were from the battle Steve had observed from the gunship.

War in the delta was escalating. The trickle of injuries became a steady flow, but the next few days provided only a taste of future trauma. Fortunately, our MILPHAP team was expanding.

The following morning, I was examining a boy in the clinic when Don burst through the doorway—a busload of casualties had arrived at the ER.

The scene was chaotic. Don counted 15 injured. As he completed his list, three more patients arrived—including a boy gored by a water buffalo!

USAID nurses were on the scene, directing hospital workers. Don organized triage and transport as corpsmen obtained supplies and assisted with the wounded. Although the carnage was horrific, it was gratifying to see Vietnamese and Americans working side by side. Within a few hours, order had been restored and the most urgent cases stabilized. Work continued until 7:00 p.m. Bill assumed evening call and Dr. Vinh invited me to his home for a special treat—fresh coconut worms, or "con tuon cha la," a VN delicacy. I successfully refused his generous offer. Perhaps another time.

Coconut worms are beetles, which lay eggs in coconut and palm trees. The Vietnamese dish consists of consuming living, wiggling larvae covered with a spicy sauce.

Most of the injured patients remained in the hospital. Those with minor wounds had been discharged. Discharged is a misnomer—patients simply walked out when they felt well or believed nothing else could be done. There were no deaths overnight.

At noon a hot game of tennis pitted USAID nurses against the doctors. While we played, the 'bou arrived with mail, supplies, and our new MILPHAP physician: Dr. Jim Jones.

Jim stepped off the Caribou to embark on his MILPHAP duties. A man of average build in his early 30s, Jim was probably 5'10" tall, with receding hairline and dark brown, penetrating but compassionate eyes and a slight stoop. He was an accomplished physician and academic, having completed Ob-Gyn residency as well as advanced training in endocrinology with impressive research projects and several scientific publications. Prior to entering the Army, he was a faculty member at the University of California San Francisco. Despite these accolades, he was an open, even humble individual who mingled easily with officers and EMs. He was assigned a hooch and deposited his gear, but within minutes was called to help Dr. Vinh in surgery. After two long operations he returned for dinner, tired, but satisfied with his first day at Bac Lieu.

On December 19 we hosted the country's minister of health, a considerable honor for Dr. Vinh. The visit was as amusing as it was memorable. In preparation, Vinh instructed hospital workers to scrub floors, clean wards, and chase animals from the wards. At the appointed hour, Don and I drove to the airport to find four individuals waiting on the runway. One was pacing in an agitated state—the minister; a small man of approximately 35 years, wearing army jungle boots and fatigues, puffing on a cigarette. He was rapidly dictating orders to his secretary, a young girl struggling to keep up with his words and his strides. Two USAID officials stood nearby, looking on with amusement.

Don apologized for being late. The officers told us they caught an earlier flight from Saigon and were 20 minutes ahead of schedule. Without notice the minister jumped in our jeep and urged Don to proceed as his secretary scrambled into the rear of the vehicle.

The administrators boarded a USAID car. Throughout our brief ride to the hospital the minister continued to dictate in a loud, affirmative voice.

We met Vinh who conducted a brief tour of the hospital. It was a colorful spectacle. The minister dominated the scene, striding confidently through the wards, asking questions, inspecting beds and cabinets, as his hapless secretary scribbled notes. Dr. Vinh remained respectful and silent. Throughout this performance I had one positive observation: the minister seemed to be genuinely interested in our deficiencies, including plumbing, electrical wiring, and the pitiful state of the buildings. Dr. Vinh remained quietly acquiescent but looked hopeful.

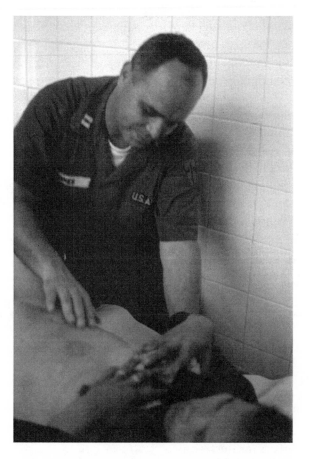

Dr. Jim Jones examining a patient with typhoid.

After the tour, we assembled in the office where the group was served orange soda pop. A folder with hospital statistics was presented to the minister, who quickly glanced at the data and then presented his conclusions and criticisms delivered in a forceful manner. The MILPHAP team sat in silence as the minister spoke rapidly in Vietnamese. His comments were brief, and the meeting ended abruptly as the minister rose, shook everyone's hand, and left the room. We were again in the jeep for our return to the airport where a Beechcraft waited with engines running. As the plane was loaded, I spoke to the Americans from USAID who told me the minister was new in office and was previously a pharmacist in a northern province. Although abrupt, he was obviously dynamic and appeared to be well motivated. With these brief comments, the ministerial visit was over. As we returned to the hospital Don and I agreed the active little man from Saigon would effect little change in Bac Lieu's facilities.

We held a team meeting, including the USAID nurses. I introduced Jim and praised the group for their efforts during the recent mass casualty. Perhaps I was too melodramatic, but everyone seemed to appreciate my comments and acknowledged the cooperative effort with their VN counterparts.

Later that morning Jim assisted Bill Owen on Ward 4, proving he was no ivory-tower intellectual, treating scabies, worms, diarrheas, and pneumonias, followed by an enthusiastic afternoon clinic. Jim also found time to give useful advice on postoperative patients.

Vinh again invited me to sample "a worm or two" at his home. I successfully countered the offer, claiming I had a Vietnamese lesson with Co Anh.

Bill Owen and the team flew to Gia Rai where they immunized more than 250 people in a MEDCAP clinic. Don's purchase of 100 piastres of candy ensured the visit's success. Candy was distributed to kids along with the vaccine. That evening Jim admitted a young boy with tetanus who died within minutes. Later, I was called to the ER by a note which simply read: Coma. However, the child was dead. The sobbing mother bundled the child and departed into the night and an uncertain future.

I gave Co Phung a tiny metal Christmas tree to assemble that had been sent by friends in the States. She spent the morning hanging foil, angels, and ornaments on the artificial plant, while humming to herself. She asked if she could take the tree home after the Christmas party. I couldn't refuse. Although Buddhist, she attended most of the MACV protestant services and read the Bible, as much to improve her English as learn about Christianity.

That evening we met at the nurses' house to wrap Christmas presents, joined by Co Phung, Co Anh, and Betty Wei, the Chinese girl who ran the novelty shop next to the small PX. Betty prepared a special dish—a ginger-flavored soup with dough balls. The treat is traditionally served at this time of year, the Chinese midwinter holiday. It is said if one partakes of it, he or she is assured of living to see the next midwinter holiday.

December 22 was my birthday. I bought several chit books at the Paddy Rat lounge and hosted a few rounds of drinks in the officers' club. There was no lack of takers for the free alcohol.

Morning preparations for the Christmas party were interrupted by a visit from the police chief who reported a 12-year-old boy had been arrested on the bridge over the city's canal with two claymore mines in his possession. He told the police additional mines had been planted and set to detonate during the holiday. Although their location was not revealed, it was suspected they were on hospital grounds. Vinh was very agitated and ordered a search of the area. The mines were never found.

The police returned a few hours later with another unpleasant announcement. A four-year-old boy had been missing for the past several days. His parents lived in a shack adjacent to the hospital. Meanwhile, the nurses had noted an offensive smell of hospital water. A manhunt ensued which ultimately led to the large cement cistern beneath the hospital kitchen. When the trap door to the cistern was opened, we were overcome with a disgusting odor and horrible sight. The bloated body of the missing child was floating in the water. Somehow the boy had gained access to the cistern and drowned. The event soured the holiday spirit and hospital staff were visibly shaken. No one was particularly hungry at supper. That night I assisted Vinh with surgery and his gallows humor was in full play. Peering over glasses above his surgical mask he quipped, "For the past few days we've all been drinking baby soup."

Christmas Eve—hospital duties were light, and at 10:00 a.m. we drove to the Catholic orphanage to deliver clothing and food. By early afternoon everyone assembled in the MILPHAP office to distribute gifts for children on the wards and hospital staff. The nurses had arranged a numbering system to ensure everyone would collect an appropriate gift. The plan worked well, although mid-way into distribution the numbering system broke down. But everyone received a present and the event was a success.

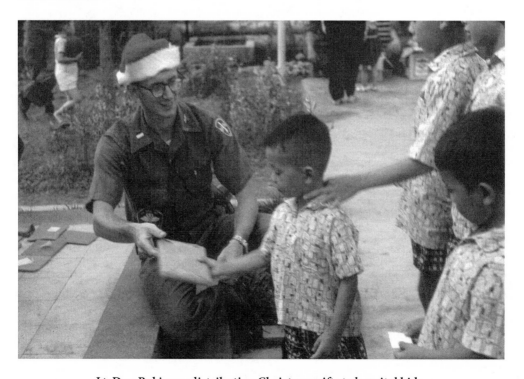

Lt. Don Robinson distributing Christmas gifts to hospital kids.

That evening the hospital generator started and we feared a surgical case was eminent. But Vinh had workers erect an array of Christmas lights to illuminate the hospital gate. Everyone applauded the multicolored spectacle. Later a candlelight service was held at 9:00 p.m. in the MACV chapel in lieu of the traditional midnight ceremony because of the curfew.

The compound was quiet Christmas day. Major Bloor conducted a protestant Christmas celebration and Father Minh held Catholic services. The hospital was similarly dormant. Dr. and Mrs. Vinh came to the MACV Christmas dinner, complete with turkey, stuffing, gravy, cranberry sauce, and mince pie. Vinh explained the VN term for holiday is "ngay le" and Christmas is known as "Noel," from the French, or "hai muoi lam" (the 25th).

Holiday festivities ended abruptly, as a major ARVN operation was scheduled December 26. More than 30 helicopters carried troops to the U Minh Forest, a VC stronghold. Two battalions of paratroopers were dropped. The mission was the largest of the year.

The wind was unabated for two days, bringing clouds of dust, fouling nostrils and burning the eyes. Vinh and Bill Owen flew to Can Tho for a health conference, leaving surgery quiet except for the usual litany of accidents. Meanwhile, Don and I worked on the old X-ray machine. The device had been used for fluoroscopy, but not films. The other machine remained inoperable because of wiring. We assembled film, cassettes, and fixer and connected a timer to the ancient device. By mid-afternoon we tested the equipment, making a series of exposures at various speeds. We hurried to the darkroom and waited anxiously to develop the film, reminiscent of my youth when I had a home darkroom. To our surprise and delight, some of the films were of adequate quality, the first X-rays taken at Bac Lieu for more than six months.

The military operation raged for two days but achieved little success. Steve was in the field both days and didn't return until 9:00 p.m. He told us the enemy was engaged but managed to escape with few casualties, a scenario to be repeated countless times.

Co Phung invited Bill Owen to her home to honor his service. Her father served chocolate ice cream from his store as Bill related his Bac Lieu adventures. His remarks were short but emotional as he confessed the experience had been life changing. In his quiet, humble voice he said he was grateful to have helped and had made many friends. After refreshments we watched TV on a tiny set in the Phung living room. There was one channel and hours of operation were limited to 8:00 to 10:00 p.m. Nevertheless, the family were proud of their modern electronic device.

Later Bill conducted his final evening rounds. He was anxious to return home, but reluctant to leave because of the enormous challenges facing Bac Lieu. As he visited the wards, he had a tearful parting with the Cambodian boy. Bill was an inspiration; his generosity and goodwill affected everyone.

After morning rounds Bill said goodbye to hospital staff and was given a farewell gift by Dr. Vinh, who drove him to the airport, where prolonged handshakes were exchanged. Vinh embraced Bill and spoke a few words, which I couldn't hear over the Caribou's engines. Bill walked to the plane, waved, and was gone, bound for Saigon, New Delhi, Rome, and Iowa, where a busy practice and family awaited him.

Bill Owen was a beloved resident of St. Ansgar, Iowa. Born to a physician father, he graduated from Cornell College, followed by medical school at Columbia University (1938–42), when he entered the Navy. After the war he returned to Iowa to practice medicine until 1984. He had three children with his first wife, including two who became physicians. His second wife of 27 years, Dorothy, was an RN, nurse practitioner, and Physician's Assistant. Bill did three tours of Vietnam as an AMA volunteer physician, as well as subsequent medical service in other countries (William E. Owen, MD, 1918–2002).

Shortly after returning from the airport, I was called to the ER for a patient with a "bi thuong" (wound). Three men in black pajamas surrounded the examining table where a similarly clad man reposed, a blood-stained rag covering his leg. The hospital attendants were conspicuously quiet but said the man had been shot by a soldier. I didn't ask the victim's political affiliation but kept a weather eye in the direction of his comrades. A bullet had traversed his leg below the knee. There was considerable loss of blood, but no bony damage. We took an X-ray, confirming my findings. I cleaned and sutured the wound and wrote admitting orders, fully expecting him to leave the hospital. But on evening rounds, he was in the post-op ward together with his three bodyguards.

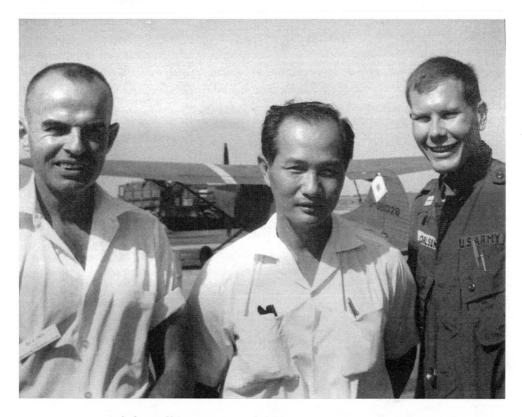

Dr. Owen's farewell at Bac Lieu airfield: Dr. Owen, Dr. Vinh, and author.

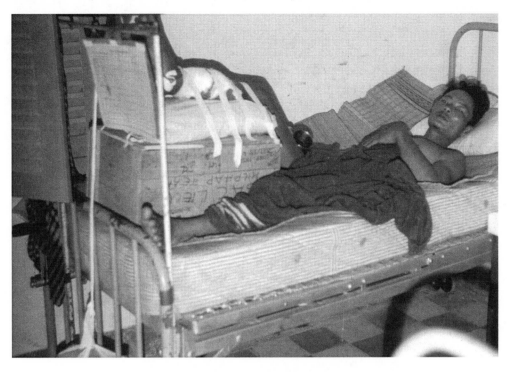

Wounded Viet Cong in hospital bed.

A snake bite victim was brought to the ER that evening. The envenomation occurred several days earlier, and the wound was badly infected. From the description, the snake may have been a krait, a very dangerous reptile. The woman had used Chinese medicines and rituals to exorcise the evil spirits instilled by the serpent. She ultimately came to the hospital because of fever and progressive swelling of her arm. Spiritualism and folk medicine dominated rural life, frequently hampering our medical efforts and frustrating Dr. Vinh, who was uniformly unsympathetic to the superstitions.

An APC (armored personnel carrier) driven by ARVN troops was hit by a VC mine buried in the roadway near the airport. The occupants were blown out of the vehicle and sustained major injuries. One soldier had traumatic amputations of both legs. Steve arranged medical evacuation to Can Tho by dust offs. I thought to myself, "We could have been the victims, as we drive that road several times a week."

Vinh's composure during an emergency was on display on the last day of the year when a routine hernia repair became a nightmare. The anesthesia machine broke down during the case, and the patient began to awaken. We struggled to restrain the semiconscious man as the anesthetist administered intravenous sedation. Throughout the crisis Vinh retained his usual placid attitude, expressing no emotion. After the crisis he removed his gown, sat on a stool, and drank an orange soda pop. Without comment or pause, he proceeded to instruct me on the multiple Vietnamese terms for "to carry." I also learned the equivalent of "one foot in the grave." Roughly translated, it means "close to the ground," or "far from the sun." In return for my lesson, I coached him on "gold," "wool," "walk," "talk," and other words with an "L," which he had difficulty pronouncing. He never ceased to amaze me.

Year's end provided a spectacular sunset, and several officers ran outside to shoot 35 mm slides. The scene was strikingly beautiful, but the poverty, filth, and disease, coupled with the horrors of the war, were omnipresent. A New Year's Eve party was held at the officers' club, although Don and I remained in our hooch with typewriter and books. There was considerable drinking.

The final months of 1966 presaged greater fighting the coming year. In September, the 11th Armored Cavalry initiated operations in 111 Corps, and marines carved out a permanent but oft-besieged base at Khe Sanh. In the delta, the 21st Division conducted multiple military campaigns with varying success. VC were resourceful and their intelligence was superior to ours. Bac Lieu would not be spared.

Chapter Sources

Jason B. Harris, Regina C. LaRocque, Firdausi Qadri, et al. "Cholera." *Lancet* 379, no. 9835 (2012): 2466–76.
Stephen W. Lacey. "Cholera: Calamitous Past, Ominous Future." *Clinical Infectious Diseases* 20, no. 5 (1995): 1409–19.
Jean-Pierre Raufman. "Cholera." *American Journal of Medicine* 104, no. 4 (1998): 386–94.
John Snow. *On the Mode of Communication of Cholera.* London: John Churchill, 1849.
David L. Swerdlow and Allen A. Ries. "Cholera in the Americas: Guidelines for the Clinician." *JAMA* 267, no. 11 (1992): 1495–99.
William E. Owen. Obituary. *Madison City Globe Gazette* (IA), July 31, 2002.

6

January 1967

MDs, Mudfish, and Monkey Brains

New Year's celebrations continued far into the night, resulting in a nearly deserted mess hall on January 1. Those who struggled to breakfast were content with coffee heavily laced with aspirin.

At noon Col. Maddox greeted junior officers in the classic New Year's Day Army tradition. MACV staff presented themselves to the commanding officer in their best uniforms as refreshments were served in the mess hall. General Minh and other dignitaries were present.

Warm weather continued. Don and I attempted to capture a small frog that entered our hooch. We didn't find the frog, but killed a large scorpion lurking behind my bunk.

On January 2, the compound resumed normal activity and Steve participated in a MEDCAP visit to the "Chieu Hoi" (open arms) repatriation camp. The government paid the former VC a bonus and provided a small subsistence allowance if they remained in their assigned quarters. On the edge of town approximately 15 Chieu Hoi families lived in a two-room shanty. Steve ran sick call and distributed food and medicines and vaccinated residents. The Chieu Hoi, or Chu Hoi, program allowed Viet Cong to repatriate to the government without penalty. Defection was facilitated by leaflets dropped from aircraft and loudspeakers. Safe conduct passes were issued, although defectors were occasionally shot. Many Chieu Hoi were successfully used in psy-war campaigns and to encourage additional defections, but VC reprisals and assassinations affected the program. Approximately 100,000 Chieu Hoi were repatriated, some of whom were successfully integrated into ARVN units.

Two AMA volunteer physicians arrived on the morning 'bou to replace Bill Owen. Our team was fortunate to have at least one VPVN doctor throughout the year, generously supplied by USAID. The latest arrivals were Dr. Ronald Passafaro, an internal medicine specialist from New York, and Dr. Lois Visscher, of Evanston, Illinois, but posted to India for the preceding 20 years as a Methodist medical missionary. Ron was a tall, large-framed man with a big smile, greying hair, and a firm handshake. When asked why she had come to Vietnam, the soft-spoken, matronly Lois responded, "I go where I am most needed." She reminded me of the female missionary in C. S. Forester's novel *The African Queen*.

Lois was a medical missionary throughout her adult life. She graduated with

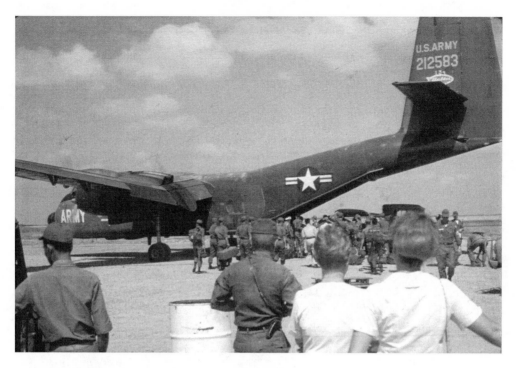

The arrival of the morning Caribou.

honors from the University of Illinois College of Medicine and completed residencies in Obstetrics, Surgery and Pediatrics, a significant accomplishment for a woman in the 1930s. She served in India as a medical missionary and was the first female to be accepted in the AMA volunteer physicians' program, returning for a second tour in 1972 as well as missionary efforts in Africa, Thailand, and an Indian reservation in Wyoming (Lois H. Visscher, MD, 1914–2002).

Ron was an internal medicine specialist who practiced in Fredonia, New York. He graduated from medical school in New York, completed training at the E. J. Meyer Memorial Hospital, and ran an active medical practice from 1952 to 1992. During World War II he was a bombardier in the Army Air Force. He was married for 54 years, with three sons and two daughters, and was prominent in many local civic and religious organizations (Ronald Passafaro, MD, 1925–2006).

We loaded the doctors' luggage in the jeep and drove to the nurses' home where Dr. Visscher would be quartered. Ron would bunk with USAID personnel.

That afternoon I gave the new physicians a tour of the hospital. Ron was stunned by the squalid conditions of the facility, whereas Lois didn't seem fazed, as she had worked under primitive medical situations for many years. As we concluded our tour, we met Dr. Vinh, who politely inquired of their backgrounds. As the customary orange soda pop was served, Vinh sized up the new arrivals and repeated his usual question to new doctors: "What do you think of Bac Lieu?"

I oriented Dr. Visscher to Wards 9 and 12, helping her learn patients and medications, and meet the VN nurses. She quickly adapted to the routine and launched into work without pause. Despite his initial reaction to the hospital, Ron was a welcome addition. He made several diagnoses that had puzzled us and finished clinic in record time.

Over drinks in the Paddy Rat Lounge I chatted with Pete Peterson, the USAID agricultural advisor. A ruddy, bourbon-drinking Texan, Pete was formerly with the Texas Department of Agriculture. He told me January is the season to harvest rice in the delta, a dangerous but profitable time of year. The peasants worked in the paddies during the long, hot days, gambling they would not be mistaken for VC by American aircraft, or VC wouldn't shoot them in their exposed position. Rice was harvested by hand, wrapped into bundles, which were carried to roads or canals by family members or buffalo. The product was dried, thrashed, packed into bags, and transported to Can Tho or Saigon. Rice was processed using ancient methods that maintained the outer covering, preventing Beri-Beri or thiamine deficiency.

Pete explained VN farmers typically yielded 2 metric tons (one metric ton = 2200 pounds) of rice per hectare, or 2.47 acres. In the United States, a farmer would lose money with such a limited crop. Yield in the States was more than twice that amount, but American farmers enjoyed controlled irrigation, fertilizer, improved seeds, and mechanization. The Vietnamese farmer depended on natural irrigation, with little or no fertilizer, and his crop was frequently bathed in salt water several months a year, inhibiting growth. Finally, VN produced one crop per year; two or more were common in the States.

Pete said he and his USAID colleagues aimed to improve farming methods, as well as import new strains of rice. USAID entrusted the military to ensure crops were protected, as VC commonly seized shipments or confiscated rice stores. Many incidents occurred at canal blocks—an aquatic roadblock. These activities were a major source of funds and food for the VC. But Pete admitted ARVN units were usually helpless to disrupt VC banditry. Canal blocks and attempts to destroy them would become an ongoing saga.

I observed my two-month anniversary in Vietnam. The interval had passed quickly. Daily events could be exciting and often frustrating, but always educational. The medical and public health challenges were overwhelming and the hospital grossly inadequate for its task, but I was optimistic we could complete some building projects. The team had been introduced to war's trauma, but we would behold much worse, hampering our efforts for meaningful progress.

The next day Joan and I reviewed plans with Dr. Vinh for the new outpatient clinic as we adapted the existing facility for Dr. Passafaro. Meanwhile, Jim planned for Dr. Visscher to help Dr. Tot on Ward 6. The only areas of the hospital with no American coverage were Dr. Khoung's wards. Neither our team or the prior group had managed to achieve any progress with the devious Khoung. His reputation was tainted, and he jealously guarded access to his territory. Joan and Linda worked on his wards and reported terrible sanitary conditions and daily breaches of medical practice. It wasn't clear why Vinh could not displace the incompetent doctor, but Khoung had been a fixture for many years and hospital politics remained opaque.

The marines landed in the delta! Military radio reported a major assault force, with elements of the 9th marine unit coming ashore near the mouth of the Co Chien river, about 15 miles from Soc Trang. Operation Deckhouse Five included U.S. and

South Vietnamese marines. It wasn't clear how this would affect the balance of power, as no other U.S. forces were in the delta. We were unaware of the fierce battles in 1–111 corps to the north where American forces were encountering heavy resistance from VC and North Vietnamese soldiers. That afternoon I saw a squadron of B-52s flying west to bomb Laos and Cambodia, and the evening was disrupted by the howitzers blasting the local countryside. The fusillade was very loud, but fortunately ended by 11:00 p.m.

Dr. Visscher accompanied the chaplain on his Sunday tour of the delta, stopping at several outposts for religious services. The circuitous flight provided Lois a good view of the region. In the afternoon Dr. and Mrs. Vinh led a caravan of vehicles to a nearby Cambodian Buddhist temple reportedly built 200 years ago. The site resembled an Oriental postcard, with tile roofs, cement dragons, multiple altars, shrines, and Buddhas, as well as frescos depicting religious scenes. We snapped pictures and posed with the monks in their saffron robes. The temple was situated on the banks of a small canal and the monks demonstrated how they caught "mud fish." When the tide receded, smaller canal tributaries drained, leaving fish stranded in the mud. The monks trudged in bare feet through the slime to collect their next meal.

We climbed into our vehicles and drove to the next point of interest—the Vietnamese Buddhist temple, a modern building in downtown Bac Lieu, where we were served tea by smiling monks, most of whom were in their early 20s. The contrast with the Cambodian temple was striking.

That evening we received seven casualties from Long My, 40 km northwest of the city. All victims were women and children wounded by bombs from aircraft.

The new AMA doctors settled into the hospital routine. Dr. Passafaro conducted adult clinic and staffed the wards as Dr. Visscher assisted Vinh on surgical cases and supervised other services.

Following the morning surgery schedule Vinh invited us to his office to share orange soda pop as he related some features of life in Vietnam. He was in a

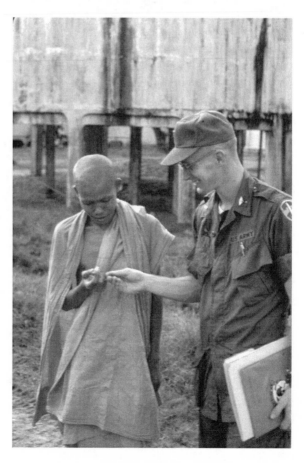

Buddhist monk and Lt. Don Robinson.

philosophic but solemn mood. He began, "The French had a saying about my people, and unfortunately, it is true: 'If the Vietnamese plant a tree, they won't water it; if they buy a dog, they won't feed it; and when they have children, they don't discipline them.'"

He shook his head and admitted many Vietnamese, even hospital workers, match the parable, lacking a sense of responsibility and purpose. Although they show concern for patients, it doesn't extend to improving conditions. He said workers smile curiously as we struggle to upgrade the facilities, believing we are fools. He sighed, "Perhaps we expect too much. We strive for their unwanted betterment and are discouraged by their laissez faire attitude." Vinh looked away for a moment, gathering his thoughts, then offered his sober assessment a similar attitude applied to the nation. He reminded us Vietnam had been at war for 25 years and previously exploited by 75 years of French rule. The citizens respected French culture but not colonialism. Vinh believed Vietnam's progress to democracy was slow, painstaking, and not assured of success. Aside from modern innovations in large cities, most Vietnamese lived a simple agrarian life, little changed for a century. He was not optimistic of a groundswell for democracy. The American dollar and military influence were strong, but he concluded it would be many years before Vietnam would catch up with the rest of the world. Unless a sense of nationalism, pride, and responsibility were created, the nation's future was uncertain. The VC had fierce determination and a sense of purpose, lacking by many who supported the government. But Vinh was appalled by the VC's unending violence and atrocities. "Why do they kill their fellow citizens?" he asked. He admitted some of the VC's tactics were to counter the overwhelming technical superiority of the United States, but how could one excuse the senseless slaughter? Despite the horror inflicted by the enemy, Vinh was not sanguine that Saigon, and its American ally would prevail.

We were shocked by his comments. Sensing our dismay and disappointment, he made a quick plea for greater efforts to help the people and for hospital improvements, finished his drink, and walked out of the office to a waiting car. We sat in stunned silence.

That evening Jim and I concluded if Vinh had such concerns for his country, we should take heed. As I typed my thoughts that night, it was difficult to capture Vinh's words, but his comments were alarming, and shattered many concepts I had held.

These were the first expressions of Vinh's views of the war, but in the forthcoming months I became privy to more of his ruminations. I remained perplexed by his comments of his countrymen. He maintained a dedication to our mutual goals, but privately was pessimistic. The war continued for nearly a decade, but his ominous predictions were prescient.

The marines pursued fighting in the delta, although they met little resistance. When faced with superior forces, the VC blended into the countryside and became invisible. They picked their battles.

Drs. Douglas and Marsh flew from Can Tho to assess our renovation projects. Douglas had been a project VN doctor with the AMA, returning as a USAID administrator. Like Col. Moncrief, Marsh was on loan to USAID from the military. Both physician-administrators represented the best of USAID and were dedicated to building civilian health care in Vietnam, despite the obstacles.

Jim developed several innovations on the pediatric ward, Trai 4. Linda, Co Anh, and Spc. Andy Anderson painted walls and purchased toys for a playroom, and Jim devised a croup tent, although we quickly ran out of oxygen. Painting and clean up continued, but the strain of work was evident on Jim's face.

I planned to give Jim a few days' rest in Saigon and to have him devote more time in maternity where his expertise could be better utilized. Jim and I were beginning to bond. As we chatted in his hooch that evening, he told me he envisioned a special project for maternity. I was curious but did not press him for details.

Vinh and I took a chopper to Phuoc Long for an update on the hamlet's clinic. During our visit the local outpost was resupplied with ammunition and food. Our Huey made a brief stop at Vinh My en route. We buzzed the landing zone, a cleared space adjacent to a rice paddy surrounded by RFPF troops. The pilot came in "hot" at 80 knots and 10 feet above the paddy. The door gunners adjusted their weapons as a precaution. We had barely touched down when one passenger scrambled off and another boarded as the crew tossed supplies from the doors. Within seconds we were skimming the tops of paddies, gaining altitude for the trip to Phuoc Long, a small village on the banks of a large canal. The area was not secure, and ARVN radio reported a company-sized unit of VC nearby. We made another hasty landing and jumped off. Ammunition and other gear were unloaded as the ship's rotors turned.

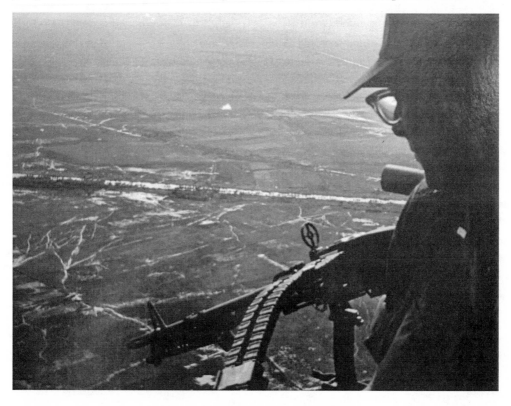

Huey gunship flying over the delta.

The Phuoc Long dispensary was housed in a cement building near the canal. Dr. Vinh said the former employee had been drafted three months ago. The remaining staff were a midwife and two maids. Most equipment had been lost or stolen, and the only surgical instruments were two rusty pairs of scissors and one hemostat. Three postpartum women reclined on mats in one of the rooms. Vinh promised the anxious midwife he would resupply the site as soon as possible and recruit another health worker.

During the return flight to Bac Lieu, I reflected on Vinh's difficult, frustrating task to administer the province's health system, running the hospital and its only surgeon. His recent sobering comments echoed in my thoughts. How did he maintain his dedication?

We constantly struggled with electrical and plumbing problems of the 60-year-old hospital. The autoclave had been repaired by a USAID mechanic, but quickly blew a fuse and Mariana and the surgical technicians were forced to light "the monster," a gasoline fired sterilizer. We were in the next room when a minor explosion resulted from a sudden release of pressure from a safety valve. Hot water and steam engulfed the room. Vinh poked his head through the door as the hissing ceased. Mariana shrugged her shoulders and raised her hands in exasperation. He walked to the blackboard and scrawled the words, "sanh nghe tu nghiep." Roughly translated it meant you die by your profession. He proposed, "A soldier dies by a bullet; a policeman at the hands of a thief; and a nurse by an exploding autoclave." We shared a good laugh, but everyone retained a healthy respect for "the monster."

Dr. Visscher accompanied Steve on a MEDCAP to two hamlets, immunizing more than 400 individuals. MEDCAPS offered the worst medical care by U.S. standards, but provided immunization for rural areas. Medicine had become a powerful political weapon.

Jim, Passafaro, and I sampled some Vietnamese fare at an open-air restaurant where we were served "trai vu sua," or "breast's milk," a purple melon in the shape of a breast with a sweet interior. The following day we all suffered gastrointestinal consequences. GI distress with diarrhea had become a frequent event for most of us. I chided myself for eating raw fruit on the local market. Fortunately, the episode was brief, and we recovered by noon, but it was a reminder of the poor sanitation throughout Bac Lieu.

A delegation of officials from Saigon arrived to dedicate the new Red Cross building. Dr. Vinh practiced his speech as Co Phung prepared an English translation. Dignitaries included Swiss and American Red Cross personnel, the chairman of the Vietnamese Relief organization, and several USAID doctors. The dedication occupied the morning, complete with band music and flag waving. There were several speeches followed by the familiar lunch with cognac. Food, blankets, and clothing were distributed by high school students.

The compound was deserted for a two-day ARVN operation near Vi Granh. A large VC unit with many prisoners was discovered and ARVN troops engaged the enemy. One of the massive Chinook helicopters was struck by ground fire, crashing with the loss of six crew members. Before retreating, VC killed 40 of their prisoners.

The VC were ruthless and obviously did not heed the Geneva Convention. I was reminded of Dr. Vinh's comments of VC atrocities.

Thoughts of the senseless slaughter prompted me to look up appropriate quotes for the evening. Plato said, "Only the dead have seen the end of war." Albert Camus wrote in *The Fall*, "The earth is dark, cher ami, the coffin thick, and the shroud opaque."

As I typed, offshore naval guns created a distant rumble echoed by the ARVN 105s. Thousands of miles away President Johnson delivered the State of the Union Address, admitting the war was far from over as he requested a record budget to fund the conflict.

The following day six casualties were brought from Vi Tranh, scene of the recent bloody fighting. All were young men with bullet or shrapnel injuries. There was no need to ask political affiliations, their eyes beheld their angst and fear. Steve helped me with a man shot in the groin. Both testicles and his penis were involved, and we were forced to sacrifice his testicles to control bleeding. The man appeared to realize we were trying to help him, although I recalled earlier times when castration was common during war. I hoped he would not blame us for his sterile condition and tried to clear my conscience with the thought ARVN castrated him—I merely completed the job.

Army radio repeated the horrors of the recent events. The breakfast table buzzed with tales of the fighting. A few officers wagered Col. Maddox would mount an operation to hunt down the VC responsible for the murder of so many prisoners. Captain Needham told me the victims did not have a chance. VC tied the prisoners to posts, machine gunned them, and threw the bodies into ditches. As they fled, hand grenades were tossed into the ditches for good measure. The butchery was difficult to comprehend.

The third MILPHAP physician arrived at noon: Dr. Charles Gueriera, an Ob-Gyn resident who had been drafted during his residency as had I. He hailed from Hahnemann Medical Center in Philadelphia. Charlie and I shared preventive medicine courses at Fort Sam Houston last summer. A slight man with curly dark hair and a ready quip, he was proud of his Italian heritage and East Coast training. His addition completed our physician group, which was complemented by our MSC officer, an expanding contingent of enlisted men, USAID nurses, and AMA volunteers.

I do not know if other teams were as well staffed, but I suspect USAID recognized the merits of supporting Dr. Vinh. Bac Lieu was fortunate to have three MILPHAP physicians throughout the year as well as a steady stream of AMA doctors. When illness reduced our numbers, additional physicians were made available, with promise of further replacements if needed. The services of the four USAID nurses were an immense aid. In addition, Steve Reynard generously gave his time, bolstering our medical manpower. I was grateful his Army superiors permitted Steve's moonlighting duties in addition to his MACV work. Our MILPHAP corpsmen were invaluable and functioned with the VN staff despite language and cultural barriers.

January 18 was the Buddha's birthday. The hospital closed at mid-day and clinics were abbreviated. ER visits included lacerations, auto and bicycle accidents, and misadventures typical of a U.S. holiday.

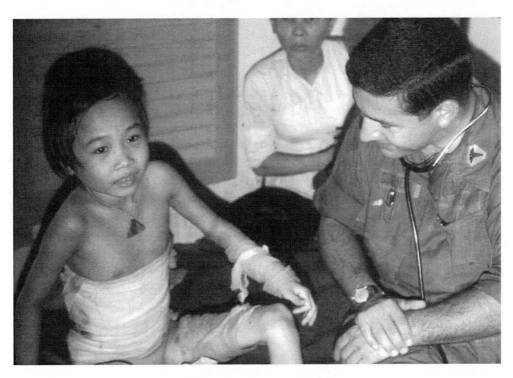

Burned girl and her mother, with Dr. Charles Gueriera.

Jim scored a big success in the maternity ward, successfully delivering healthy twins from a mother with severe toxemia of pregnancy. The midwives had given the woman up for dead.

Jim, Passafaro, and Vinh flew to Saigon for a much-needed weekend of unofficial R&R. Meanwhile, the weather had cooled to a comfortable 60 degrees, prompting hospital workers to complain, "Lanh qua" (very cold).

With three physicians absent, co-chiefs Charlie and I performed surgery and staffed wards and clinics. He admitted a patient with tetanus, a young boy who was allergic to the antitoxin. The boy came to the hospital late in the illness' course and had difficulty breathing. He died two days later.

Phuoc Long was mortared, yielding five injured as we learned of an American air strike near Soc Trang that killed and wounded a score of civilians. A company-size group of VCs fired at aircraft from a highly populated region. The counterfire from the gunships was devastating. Once again, citizens were caught between VC and the Americans. A major who witnessed the scene said it was horrific. His description matched a column I read in the *Chicago Tribune* by John Steinbeck:

> We and our allies too often kill and injure innocent people in carrying out a military operation. The VC invariably wash themselves with innocents. They set up a machine gun in the doorway of a peasant's house and herd the children close around it, knowing our reluctance to return fire at the cost of people. They build their bunkers in thickly populated areas for the same reason. And people do get hurt. I've seen the care we take to avoid it, and instant care when it cannot be helped.... I find I have no access to the thinking of the wanton terrorist.

Why do they destroy their own people, their own poor people, whose freedom is their verbal concern? Can anyone believe that the VC who can do this kind of thing to their own people would be concerned for their own welfare if they had complete control? I find I can't.

As our colleagues enjoyed Saigon, Charlie and I developed GI symptoms prompted by another trip to a downtown restaurant. Fortunately, the hospital was quiet. I lay in my hooch, giving myself injections of an antiemetic and forcing down paregoric to a rebellious stomach. Our symptoms heralded another episode of acute gastroenteritis due an acute viral infection.

Diarrheal illness is the world's most common infectious disease, causing as many as five billion cases yearly. Noroviruses are the primary culprit. General Neel wrote, "The most common disease among U.S. soldiers in VN was diarrhea ... the greatest number of cases was sporadic and caused by a breakdown in sanitation or eating locally procured vegetables." Fortunately, more serious GI disorders such as cholera or typhoid were virtually unknown among U.S. personnel.

Jim and Ron returned from a busy holiday. They were wined and dined by Vinh and sampled Saigon's night life, dancing with young women in *áo dàis* in a Cholon nightclub before curfew terminated the night's entertainment. The outing was a much-needed break for Jim who resumed work with enthusiasm. He now oversaw the maternity ward.

More rain and fog. The MACV surgeon general, Col. Eisner was scheduled to visit Bac Lieu, but bad weather grounded flights. Steve also luckily cancelled his trip. His 'bou made it aloft but received heavy ground fire and returned to the field. When the aircraft landed more than 20 bullets were discovered in the fuselage. Fortunately, no one was injured, and the plane remained flight capable.

Another child in the ER died as I began my exam. It is unnerving to have a patient succumb as you place your stethoscope on its chest. The cause the death was unknown, possibly pneumonia. Between sobs, the mother said the boy had a cough and fever. The distraught family wrapped the child in a blanket and carried him down the ER steps. I asked Mr. Ky, our interpreter, if the family could afford a funeral. He replied soberly, "They are very poor—they will take the baby home and dig a hole behind their hut. Funerals are very expensive." That afternoon I saw workmen preparing a coffin near the morgue. Coffins for the wealthy were made of hardwood—varnished and painted mahogany and teak. Wood was expensive, and funeral processions, complete with trumpets, drums, and professional mourners, costly. The rich were buried above ground, with cement catafalques; the poor returned to the earth.

The compound buzzed with news from a local outpost. Either VC attacked or, more likely, ARVN personnel became drunk and tossed grenades at one another. Twelve casualties were evacuated to Can Tho.

I received a call from USAID of a suspected case of smallpox in Phuoc Long. Smallpox is a deadly, contagious disease and vaccination in VN was incomplete in the 1960s.

Smallpox, or *Variola*, is a life-threatening infection by a DNA virus that is large enough to be seen with a light microscope. The term "variola" dates to AD 570, when a Catholic bishop borrowed the word from the Latin "spotted or pimple." Many

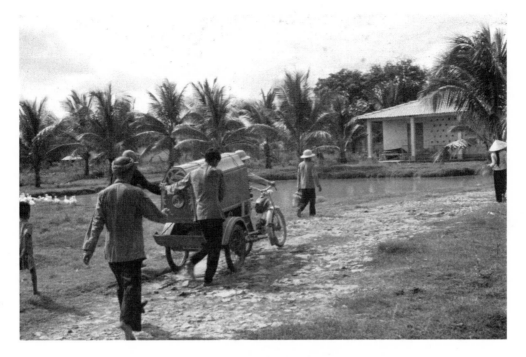

Coffin en route to hospital morgue.

assume that smallpox was the basis for the famous line: "A pox o' your throat" from Shakespeare's *The Tempest*, although the phrase probably referred to syphilis, "The Great Pox."

The disease has been known since antiquity and Egyptian mummies including Ramses V exhibited typical facial pox lesions. Children are disproportionally affected and account for up to 90 percent of cases.

We usually assume vaccination began with Edward Jenner's inoculation experiment of a British milkmaid infected with cowpox. But "variolation" had been utilized for centuries in China, India, and Africa. In colonial America, the Reverend Cotton Mather advocated the technique, and it was common knowledge if one recovered from smallpox, he was protected. Transmission of the disease is by person-to-person or via fomites such as clothing or other items. Smallpox may have been the first biological weapon, as infected blankets were reportedly given to American Indians by British troops during the revolutionary and Indian wars.

Intensive efforts at eradication were made in the 1960s and 1970s. In 1967 more than 40 countries reported smallpox, including Vietnam, and we were obliged to investigate the patient in Phuoc Long. The last wild case of smallpox was seen in 1977, and the disease declared eradicated in 1980. No U.S. personnel in VN were infected. Despite this false alarm, we saw no smallpox in Bac Lieu.

A helicopter took Don and me to Phuoc Long, along with Dr. Visscher, as she had seen smallpox in India. Like most U.S. physicians, I'd only read about the terrible disease. When we arrived, we were taken to the potential patient, a 13-year-old Cambodian boy. He was walking and playing with other children. It soon became apparent the history differed from what had been reported, as the boy and his parents only spoke Cambodian. He appeared well and exam did not reveal serious illness or skin lesions. We excluded the diagnosis but vaccinated 150 villagers.

Phuoc Long, site of the suspected smallpox patient, was attacked with several casualties. Victims slowly trickled to Bac Lieu for two days.

Stars and Stripes newspaper listed 147 American deaths in VN the prior week, a significant increase from even two months earlier. The article also reported 475,000 U.S. troops were currently in Vietnam, substantially more than the Korean war.

Dr. Vinh was in a playful mood after surgery. He took delight describing particularly unappetizing dishes to his American guests such as coconut worms. Today's topic was "an oc khi" (monkey brain). He informed us the traditional Chinese delicacy was still available in Cholon. Guests are seated around a circular table into which 4" holes have been bored. Live monkeys are placed under the table, and a monkey's head is positioned at each hole. Vinh continued the story in a particularly gruesome fashion, relishing in our disgust as he embellished his remarks, concluding with an offer to sample the dish during our next visit to Saigon. Vinh was amused by our responses. Co Phung later told us the practice existed but was only of historical interest.

In the afternoon Jim demonstrated a simplified technique of circumcision to midwives and Dr. Tot. Jim was hopeful they would perform the procedure on more male infants, as many children suffered from phimosis, a congenital narrowing of the foreskin with scarring, difficulty urinating, and risk of infection.

Interludes of Vietnamese life competed with realities of war. As fighting in the delta accelerated, hospital tasks increasingly focused on trauma. We received victims of VC attacks and atrocities as well as casualties from ARVN military operations or U.S. aircraft. Regardless of the source, the wounded came in ever-increasing numbers. H&I salvos by the adjacent 105 mm ARVN artillery battery were now routine each evening. Life was frequently interrupted by violence.

The day began calmly, as Vinh offered to take us to a cockfight behind the police chief's house that afternoon. Cockfighting was popular, with heavy betting. Steve and I were in the MACV dispensary, deciding if we would make any wagers on the roosters.

A tremendous explosion shook the compound. Seconds later Steve's phone rang, and he learned a bomb had been detonated at a subsector station downtown. He grabbed his medical bag and ran to his post as I hurried to the hospital.

From the rear gate I saw taxis, cyclos, pedicabs, and ARVN jeeps proceeding to the hospital, honking horns, ringing bells, with yelling drivers as they maneuvered the rutted road to the entrance. The scene was almost comical, with a bizarre array of makeshift ambulances. But it was no comedy—the trail of blood left by the vehicles and their maimed and lifeless occupants told a sorrowful story.

The ER was bedlam—thirty-odd patients reposed on beds, stretchers, and the floor, as relatives, soldiers, and inquisitive children crowded the room. Family members walked from bed to bed, searching for a friend or relative. One woman with a gaping head wound died as I entered. Another was bleeding profusely from an arterial injury of her leg. Charlie and Ron were desperately trying to affix a tourniquet to stem the bleeding. Dr. Visscher and the nurses arrived moments later and organized a triage system as Don and medics started IVs and transported patients to surgery.

Five casualties were in critical condition, including the woman with arterial bleeding. Two men with chest wounds died despite attempts to place chest tubes.

Vinh was in the operating room within minutes and toiled throughout the day as we took turns as his assistant.

Most of the injured were innocent bystanders who were near the building at the time of the explosion. A total of seven were killed directly or shortly thereafter; another thirty-five were transported to the hospital.

I later learned the story. The bomb had been carried to the building by two women. A guard approached them as they manipulated the bomb's controls. The women fled and seconds later the weapon exploded, digging an eight-foot crater, killing the guard and several others as it sent fragments in all directions.

One of the women who detonated the bomb was injured, allowing police to arrest her. Amazingly, she was not murdered by the mob that soon developed. Police brought her to the ER and I treated her under the careful watch of several guards. She was a plump woman of 23 years who was calm as I operated on her wounds, freely giving details to the police, apparently unconcerned of her fate. For reasons I could not recall, she was familiar to me.

Vinh took us to the site of the explosion the following morning. Workmen were filling in the crater and removing debris. The subsector's front wall was cracked and buckled, pockmarked with hundreds of shards of shrapnel. The roof had been blown off and surrounding trees had no leaves. A pagoda across the street

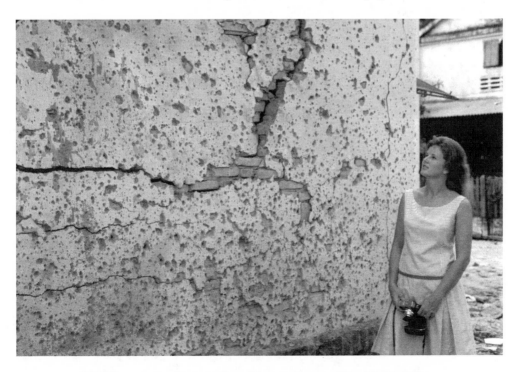

USAID nurse Pat Krebsbach and bomb-damaged Bac Lieu building.

was in shambles. Despite the carnage, life downtown appeared unaffected except for the curious.

As the city resumed its routine, the hospital also adapted and Vinh held a party for Dr. Visscher that evening. Lois would work her second month in My Tho, a province with a critical doctor shortage. Vinh was the gracious host, plying guests with food, beverages, cigarettes, and cigars. Although Dr. Visscher did not smoke or drink, she enjoyed the party. Dr. Vinh described his year in France in 1960, when he received advanced surgical training, including plastic surgery procedures. To conclude the evening, Mrs. Vinh sang opera arias as well as several Vietnamese songs, her soprano voice a contrast to the recent terrible events.

The next afternoon I drove downtown to purchase some candy for kids on the pediatric ward. I beheld a strange sight. A woman was calmly shopping, surrounded by her three children. She was "wearing" a large python around her neck and shoulders. Other shoppers were unaffected by the spectacle. Children either ignored the creature or patted it as one might greet a poodle and her owner on Hollywood boulevard. I subsequently became the owner of such a beast.

We learned the woman who detonated the bomb downtown was a MACV compound hooch girl, explaining my feeling of familiarity.

For January's final evening offshore, Naval gunfire accompanied the ARVN howitzers' pounding, as the country prepared for Tet.

Chapter Sources

C. S. Forester. *The African* Queen. London: William Heinemann, 1935.

Lois H. Visscher Papers, 1914–2002. Philadelphia, PA: Presbyterian Historical Society.

Ronald A. Passafaro. Obituary. *Buffalo News*. New York, January 10, 2006.

Roger I. Glass, Umesh D. Parashar, and Mary K. Estes. "Norovirus Gastroenteritis." *New England Journal of Medicine* 361, no. 18 (2009): 1776–85.

John Steinbeck. "Letters from John Steinbeck." *Chicago Tribune*, January 22, 1967.

Albert Camus. *The Fall*. New York: Random House, 1957.

Spurgeon Neel. "Preventive Medicine." Chapter 8 in *Medical Support of the U.S. Army in Vietnam, 1965–1970*. Washington, D.C.: U.S. Government Printing Office, 1973.

D. A. Henderson. "Epidemiology in the Global Eradication of Smallpox." *International Journal of Epidemiology* 1, no. 1 (1972): 25–30.

David A. Koplow. *Smallpox: The Fight to Eradicate a Global Scourge*. Berkeley: University of California Press, 2003.

Michael B. A. Oldstone. *Viruses, Plagues and History: Past, Present, and Future*. Oxford: Oxford University Press, 2010.

Shakespeare. *The Tempest*. Act 1, Scene 1.

7

February

Tet, Typhoid, and Tetanus

The spirit of Tet was alive and animated. Flags, banners, and posters proclaimed the coming of the new year. Vendors hawked toys, candy, and all manner of trinkets to entice young and old. Hospital census had fallen, and many patients left to be home for the holiday. The Vietnamese worked long hours, often seven days a week. But at Tet everything stopped.

Tet is the Vietnamese new year and occurs in late January or early February during the second new moon of the lunar calendar. Although similar to the Chinese New Year, the Vietnamese holiday is distinct and has been celebrated for several hundred years. It is one of the country's most important celebrations, and festivities persist for at least three days. Special foods are prepared, and families gather as individuals reflect on the past and make plans for the coming year. The burning of votive papers and offerings concludes the holiday.

During Tet of 1968 the Viet Cong and North VN launched massive and widespread attacks throughout VN, known as the General Offensive, that involved attacks on Saigon and more than 30 provincial capitals with considerable loss of life, including thousands of civilians and more than 40,000 North Vietnamese and VC troops. The U.S. and Saigon forces ultimately prevailed, but the magnitude of the offensive shocked the American public and accelerated disillusionment with the war. The offensive was also costly to the VC and conduct of the war increasingly became a North Vietnamese enterprise.

Bob Brittis replaced me as MOC of the team in late 1967 and was in Bac Lieu for the 1968 Tet offensive. Years later he recalled those terrible days. The VC planned well, and timed their attack when ARVN were off duty, at home with families, or drunk. Many soldiers had fired their ammunition in celebration or did not have their weapons. The VC commandeered a school that became their headquarters and hospital. They fired from the structure until it was ultimately destroyed by artillery. The entire town became a battleground and the MACV compound a target. No quarter was given and Bob and other MILPHAP members were fired upon. It took several days for ARVN to vanquish the VC, with considerable loss of life.

As festivities for Tet dominated Bac Lieu, Charlie took call, treating the usual cholera, pneumonias, and various diarrheal diseases plus injuries from fireworks and accidental gunshot wounds. The next morning, he and I flew to Saigon—he to check his finances, and I for laboratory tests for persistent abdominal discomfort. Saigon was hectic than usual—the roads were covered with cyclos, taxis, bicycles, dogcarts, and all manner of cars, trucks, and military vehicles.

Clouds of exhaust from Saigon's traffic mixed with the sulfur odor of sulfur of firecrackers. Charlie headed to MACV and I to the 17th Field Hospital. We met for dinner at the Rex. From the rooftop we saw flares dropped from circling planes, followed by machine gun tracers as enemy locations were located. Nearby, firecrackers

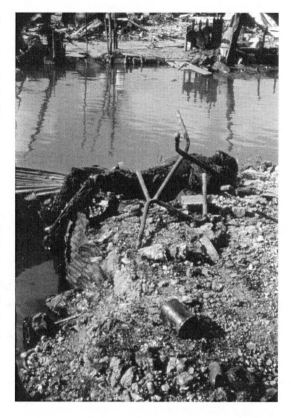

Bac Lieu damage and death from 1968 Tet offensive (unknown VN photographer, sent to author).

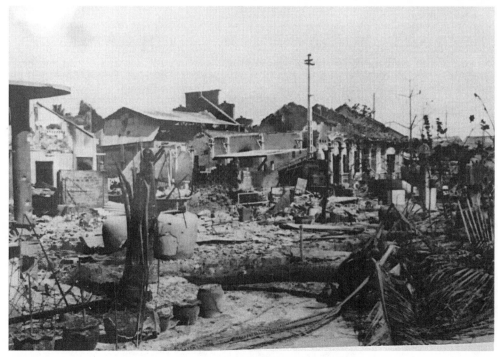

Bac Lieu destruction during 1968 Tet offensive (unknown VN photographer, sent to author).

popped and sparklers twinkled as Saigon celebrated, a unique combination of pyrotechnics.

I returned to the hospital in the morning for more tests and X-rays and caught a cyclo to the Cholon PX. The store resembled a huge supermarket on opening day. Hundreds of officers, enlisted men, government employees, and foreign troops pushed carts, clamoring to be first in line for the latest items on display. The Hi-Fi shop received the most attention. As I waited, Nancy Sinatra and her entourage were escorted through the store. Although she was an object of attention, shoppers were more concerned with their place in line.

After dinner Charlie and I walked down Tu Do Street for a drink. We were immediately set upon by tea girls. Abandoning the effort, we retreated to USAID house where I read the latest *Time* magazine. The now familiar phrase, "Winning the Hearts and Minds," had been reduced to "WHAM." Another article reported the defense budget had risen to $73 billion, most of which was slated for Vietnam.

I booked a flight to Bac Lieu and we remained at the USAID guest house for a final night, although sleep was difficult due to firecrackers, which cracked until after midnight. The barrage restarted at 6:30 a.m., together with band music and speeches from a nearby loudspeaker. As we drove to the airport a Chinese dragon danced on the sidewalk to the delight of clapping bystanders.

Our flight to Bac Lieu was delayed and Don drove us directly to the hospital in the dark. As he maneuvered around potholes, he told us several ARVN soldiers had become drunk, firing their weapons, mortars, flares, and any available incendiaries. Some of these Tet events led to injuries, but no deaths. Everyone was celebrating the new year.

We arrived as two patients were carried into the ER, a father and son who tripped a VC mine near Vinh Chau. The wounds were serious but not life threatening. I bid Charlie and Don goodnight and called to open surgery and start the generator. After a long delay, Ong Phuoc, the chief surgery technician, trotted to the building and stood in front of me with a blank stare. Suddenly he vomited, stumbled to an adjacent stretcher, and collapsed—drunk as a lord. Fortunately, Ong Tram, another OR technician, also drunk, but in somewhat better condition, arrived and prepared the OR. After operating on the father and son, I sat on the ER steps, waiting for the next patient. The pause was brief, as a bus from Gia Rai arrived, bearing a man who had attempted suicide with a razor. Miraculously, the blade missed the major vessels of the neck, but the man was bleeding profusely and had nearly transected his larynx. As I repaired the wound the inebriated surgical technician taunted the poor victim with insults and references to his ancestry.

The hospital was nearly deserted—the remaining patients were too weak to leave or dying. A child died on the pediatric ward and the mother asked the staff if the dead child could remain so she could continue her Tet celebrations.

As the holiday ended, firecrackers and other explosions became rare, and patients returned to the wards. The compound was quiet. GIs remained in their hooches, writing letters or listening to tape recorders. A military operation was scheduled for the next day. I received a reassuring call from Saigon: my lab tests for parasites or bacterial infections were negative.

The next morning Dr. Vinh escorted me to a small shack downtown surrounded by lily-covered ponds. Inside were fishbowls and fighting fish, small black and yellow creatures that attacked one another with amazing ferocity when placed together. Behind the meager shop were cages that held fighting cocks. Life was harsh in Vietnam and blood sports such as cockfighting and fish duels were popular entertainment with considerable betting.

Dr. Visscher departed for My Tho. In her absence I held Red Cross clinic with Mrs. Vinh's help, followed by a trip to the refugee center on the outskirts of town. The pitiful structure housed 20 families. Joan, Mrs. Vinh, and I distributed gifts and held sick call. I examined a boy who had been sick for several days. He was indeed ill, with signs of peritonitis. We arranged for his admission and that afternoon Vinh and I operated and found multiple intestinal perforations from typhoid. The child died a few hours later.

Typhoid was the other life-threatening intestinal infection we saw, due to the bacterium *Salmonella typhi*. Both cholera and typhoid are related to poor sanitation with fecal contamination of food or water, but the two organisms produce contrasting diseases. Unlike cholera, typhoid is an invasive infection with systemic complications. Asymptomatic carriers, so-called Typhoid Marys, may spread infection to others, but most patients develop severe intestinal inflammation with risk of perforation.

Like cholera, typhoid's cause was not identified until midway through the 19th century. Typhoid and typhus, an unrelated disease due to a bacterium known as *Rickettsia*, had been confused, and typhoid owes its name, *typhi*, to typhus, which is transmitted by lice, fleas, and mites. In the mid–19th century, British and French physicians identified the infectious nature of typhoid and finally distinguished typhus versus typhoid, or abdominal typhus as it was known. The first vaccine was produced in 1896.

Typhoid fever is fulminant, with severe abdominal pain and the risk of septic shock and multiple organ failure, which may be fatal unless antibiotics are given promptly. Intestinal perforation is a usual prelude to death. Aside from an episode of typhoid I acquired during a trip to Mexico, I had never observed the devastation produced by this organism.

Ron Passafaro accompanied Steve on a MEDCAP near Vinh Loi. They returned as several casualties arrived from Vinh Chau, scene of the massacre a day earlier. The repaired X-ray machine produced several useful images.

The attack on Vinh Chau killed 21 RFPF workers. We had been scheduled to visit the area to distribute clothing and medication but organized an alternative convoy by jeep and sampan to Vinh My. Mariana brought clothes donated by friends in Illinois. During the visit we held sick call for nearly 175 inquisitive villagers. Some were sick, others merely wanted to see the American Bac Si's.

We returned from Vinh My late in the afternoon. I yearned for an evening of rest, but was called that night to see a patient in the ER with a vexing medical problem. The woman was in panic but only her eyes mirrored the terror. She lived in a local hamlet and her family said she complained of a stiff neck for a few days but was now short of breath and having spasms. Lying on the exam table, she arched her

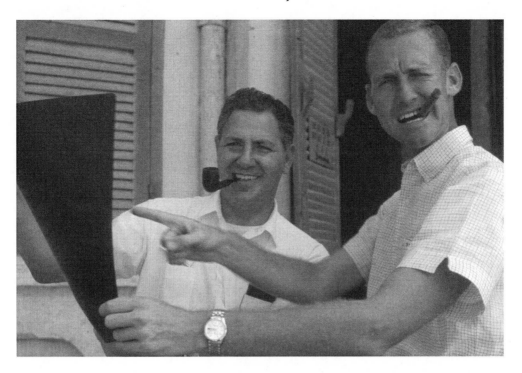

Drs. Ron Passafaro and Steve Reynard examining X-ray from the repaired machine.

back stiffly as I examined her. Her eyes were pleading but her countenance didn't display fear. In fact, she seemed to be smiling, although she could hardly breathe. What was she trying to tell me? I was puzzled. She was awake, so meningitis was not a consideration. Was she having seizures? Could this be a stroke? Was she psychotic? Suddenly, it came to me: this was tetanus. She was expressing the malevolent grin of risus sardonicus, due to contraction of her facial muscles. Unable to cough or take a deep breath, her puny respiratory efforts triggered additional muscle contractions and stridor, worsening the shortness of breath. I listened to her lungs, which confirmed pneumonia. She would die of respiratory failure from progressive spasm of her larynx or drown in her secretions. I had only read about tetanus or lockjaw, as it was rare in the U.S.

She began spitting up blood-tinged sputum and her breathing was now a continuous whine from narrowing of her larynx. I told the ER nurse she needed a tracheostomy (artificial airway) and ran to surgery to start the generator and alert the surgical crew as the pharmacy searched for antitoxin. When I reached the building, the lights were ablaze, and the generator was running full speed. Dr. Vinh was donning a scrub suit as he smoked an English cigarette. A patient was being readied for surgery, another ectopic pregnancy. Vinh greeted me in Vietnamese and I scrubbed and gowned.

We completed the surgery and Vinh departed, bidding me "bonne soirée" as he walked to his car. I hurried to the ER and prepared the woman for the neck procedure, which required much longer than it should; every movement triggered more muscle contractions. We finally established the artificial airway and her chances for survival had improved, but pneumonia could be fatal, and she would require sedation for several days.

Tetanus is a strange disease. After a wound is contaminated with *Clostridium tetani*, the bacteria produce a toxin that slowly and silently attacks the victim's muscles and nervous system. Progressive muscle contractions ensue, often including the face with "lockjaw" and the characteristic risus sardonicus expression. Until recently, tetanus was uniformly fatal from respiratory failure and pneumonia. Victims are awake throughout the course, with intense pain. Americans are immunized early in life with DPT vaccine—diphtheria, pertussis (whooping cough) and tetanus, but in the 1960s most rural residents of Vietnam had not been immunized. A trivial cut could lead to death.

The tetanus toxin is one of the most powerful natural poisons, surpassed only by that of *Clostridium botulinum*, a related bacteria. Paradoxically, the botulinum toxin does not produce spasm, but muscle paralysis. Tiny doses of botulinum toxin are now given for several medical and cosmetic indications. The hospital had a supply of tetanus antitoxin, which could be lifesaving if given early but was in limited supply and risked allergic reactions.

My father saw tetanus as a youngster in Iowa and had a healthy respect for the disease as a general practitioner. Although immunized as a toddler, my 12-year-old brother developed suspicious symptoms from a cut, which prompted my father to take him to the LA county hospital for evaluation. Keith spent a harrowing night on a ward, but no signs of tetanus developed, and he was discharged the next day. I had never encountered tetanus prior to VN.

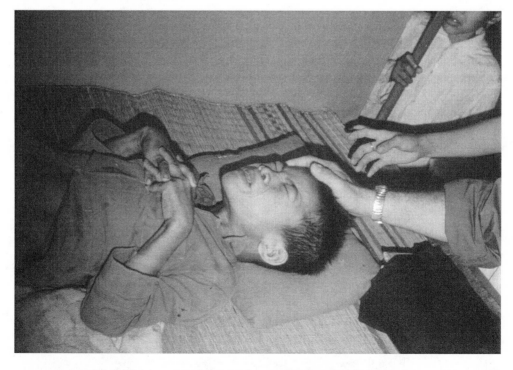

Boy with tetanus and classic risus sardonicus facial expression.

The day began with a sticky, humid, stillness that alternated with bright sunshine and the sea's breath. Clouds, low, grey, and menacing, hung over Bac Lieu throughout the day. The hospital awoke from its slumber, stretching and reluctantly receiving its first patients.

Bac Lieu was calm. We were unaware of the fierce battle in the north involving Tra Binh, a major clash involving Republic of Korea forces with thousands of combatants. A few days later the United States launched Operation Junction City, the largest airborne assault since World War II, which persisted for more than two months and led to the death of nearly 3,000 enemy. President Johnson sent a letter to Ho Chi Minh offering to suspend bombing if North Vietnam would stop sending men into South Vietnam. And on February 21, Bernard Fall, an early, prophetic observer of the war and author of *Street Without Joy*, died from injuries sustained by a landmine. Fall's book and Graham Greene's *The Quiet American* were two crucial volumes in my education of Vietnam's war.

But the events in the north were invisible to us. Our reality was the delta, as we anticipated the next VC attack or divisional operation.

Steve assisted Vinh on an amputation for gangrene. The operating room was filled with the putrid odor of the dead leg. Fortunately, other patients were doing well, including the woman with tetanus.

Miss Katherine Gallagher flew from Can Tho for a week's visit. She was a nurse anesthetist from USAID who traveled delta hospitals, teaching anesthesia to VN technicians. A plump woman with an infectious grin, she quickly befriended our anesthetists Ong Tam and Co Twi, disarming any doubts they may have had of the U.S. female instructor. She participated in several surgeries, gently providing tips to her VN colleagues in a calm and nonthreatening manner.

I examined a girl of 14 at the request of the police. She was a VC suspect and had been kept in the city jail for several weeks. She was very ill, likely from typhoid fever. The police reluctantly agreed to have her admitted and on evening rounds we saw her on the ward without guards or restraints. She glared at me as I made rounds. Other patients were either unaware of her identity or didn't particularly care. Other female VC prisoners had not fared as well. When a girl was apprehended after the recent shelling, civilians attacked and nearly killed her before the police took control. We learned the former hooch girl involved in the bombing would be executed the following month.

Residents of the MACV compound were in the field, sharing a bivouac with their Vietnamese counterparts as a large ARVN operation continued for another day. U.S. news agencies reported ongoing B-52 raids and their deleterious effects on peace talks.

Although Jim was on call, he summoned me at 3:00 a.m. to help with a woman who had been shot by the police. She had five bullet wounds that from close-range shots. The story was garbled, although the woman had failed to "pay off" officials or was the victim of jealousy. The wounds were very serious, and Jim asked Vinh to scrub on the case. No blood donors were found, although the police eventually located the husband, who gave a unit of blood. The patient's 20-year-old daughter was also brought to the ER and the unwilling girl restrained as technicians extracted a unit from her. The patient remained in shock, and Jim donated blood. During surgery Jim became light-headed, and I helped Vinh finish the procedure. One wound was abdominal, and the bullet passed through the intestine. We found a large ascaris worm in the abdomen that had exited through the path of the bullet. The operation was long and complicated. Vinh's skill and judgment were impressive. He was quick, competent, and fearless, well suited to Vietnam's conditions. I wondered how he did this day in, day out.

As Jim and I trudged to the compound in the early light of morning, we saw dozens of gunships buzzing overhead like horseflies in preparation for the day's action.

That afternoon the gunshot woman went into shock. Dr. Vinh and I donated blood, but she died at 6:00 p.m.

More bad news at dinner. We learned the 21st Division's operation was extensive, and many VC and ARVN soldiers were killed, as well as American casualties. Fighting would continue the next morning.

That evening I saw a young man with fever and abdominal pain. He was moribund when I examined him—temperature 104 degrees, with a pulse of 180 per minute and unobtainable blood pressure. Despite our efforts, he died within a few minutes. The illness was a mystery—perhaps typhoid fever. He was a respected member of a prominent family, and people soon crowded the ER, crying and wailing, creating a frustrating and depressing situation. Later we admitted another patient with tetanus, and Jim lost a little girl with meningitis. It is one thing for a doctor to admit sick patients—but crushes the mind when so many died needlessly. We were helpless to alter the outcome of many.

At least 300 VC were killed during the two-day battle, which involved two battalion-sized units of insurgents (a VN battalion includes up to 500 members). Stoney said at least 160 ARVN were wounded, plus nearly three score killed in action. Nine helicopters were downed by VC machine guns. A sergeant from the compound was killed. Steve and I had seen him in sick call a few weeks earlier. He was a handsome young man who had completed his tour of duty but extended for another six months. He was shot in the head by automatic weapons fire. What a waste.

Another EM, PFC—endured a terrifying ordeal and was lucky to survive. He was ambushed, pinpointed by machine guns from multiple sites and forced to crouch in three feet of water for several hours as bullets and mortars whizzed overhead. He was rescued after napalm was dropped on a VC machine gun nest a mere 50 yards distant. He returned to the compound that evening, dirty, weak, and glassy-eyed. What an experience for an 18 year old. When I was his age, death and killing were of no concern—occurring only in books or movies. Life was simple and beautiful. After his ordeal he would certainly view the future differently. What a stupid war. My thoughts turned to the female prisoner on the ward—consumed with hate and fear. Man is the supreme predator, excelling all animals in killing, especially the murder of his species. We have the means to accomplish our own extinction. I mused, "How long before we do so?"

Clouds hovered over the compound like smoke. Someone forgot to shut off a lavatory faucet, and there was no hot water for showers. After breakfast, Don and

I walked through the compound past the barbed wire fence and rear gate, returning the salutes of U.S. and Vietnamese guards. The VC prisoners working on the new outpatient building waved to us as white-shirted police guards squatted nearby. Work went slowly—only the Americans were in a hurry.

At lunch a rumor circulated the VC planned another attack. Our interpreters told Don they no longer wished to be picked up and driven to the hospital by jeep, preferring to walk. The rumor included the threat U.S. vehicles would be targets of terrorist action.

Don earned his second bar and became Captain Robinson. Col. Maddox officiated and awarded a silver star to Captain Stewart for heroic action. There was a memorial service for the sergeant killed during the recent operation. Following the chaplain's eulogy, "Taps" was played.

Night call was busy—kids with encephalitis, typhoid fever, several pneumonias, and a woman eight-months pregnant with severe abdominal pain. The diagnosis mystified me until she began vomiting worms.

Sunny but windy weather blew into Bac Lieu and dust was everywhere. Robert Mitchum visited the compound as part of USO's celebrity tours. I was shocked at his appearance—gaunt, with slim face and extremities, although he met with officers and EMs, chatting easily as he posed for pictures and signed autographs.

Pediatric and obstetrical emergencies occupied our day. Jim managed to obtain a blood donor for a child with severe anemia and massive enlargement of his liver and spleen. As Jim started the transfusion, the boy looked at him imploringly and via the interpreter said, "Please, Bac Si, don't let me die!" The mother's face echoed the sentiment with expressions of fear and hope. The boy likely had an underlying malignancy, possibly lymphoma, with a very poor prognosis. Not all tragedies were due to the war.

General Westmoreland, commander of all U.S. forces, visited Bac Lieu. He and General Minh met at a nearby military outpost. We were grateful for their choice of location, which did not disrupt the city.

Between surgeries, Dr. Vinh called me to discuss a political problem. The ARVN medical unit was trying to assume control of Ward 3. Vinh said Bac Si Dick, the army medical commander, had attempted to secure the ward for more than a year, although Vinh had successfully blocked the effort. But Dick had obtained a letter from the minister of health supporting his position. Vinh told me ARVN didn't need the ward and the structure had always been part of the civilian hospital. Until a new military facility was built, ARVN casualties were evacuated to Can Tho or Soc Trang. Also, the ward had been built by funds donated by a Bac Lieu businessman, whose plaque adorned one of the walls. Finally, ARVN doctors spent little time in military activities or at the adjacent medical facility and had lucrative private practices downtown. Vinh patiently explained these facts as I tried to understand the squabble. I hoped he would prevail and preserve the hospital for civilian care, but I could offer only moral support.

It was Washington's birthday. The VN didn't honor the father of our country and the hospital operated at full capacity. The compound was quiet, but the clubs were busy. That evening, a sergeant became disruptive in the EM club and was ousted by the "bouncer." The disgruntled, inebriated man returned with his .45 pistol. A scuffle ensued and the weapon fired, the bullet narrowly missing another sergeant as it spent itself in the wall. The drunken soldier was escorted to his hooch to sleep it off and face disciplinary action.

The following morning a bus discharged two injuries. An eight-year-old boy found a dud mortar shell. His mother grabbed the ordnance, but it exploded, severing the boy's right hand, and destroying his left eye. His mother sustained minor trauma. Charlie and Vinh completed the boy's amputation and removed his eye, a disheartening surgery.

Life in Bac Lieu had become semi-routine, but stress took its toll. Numbed by the endless trauma to women and children, treatment of injuries became second nature, but was always challenging and increasingly depressing. The physical damage etched emotional scars on the caregivers. One salvation was the ability to travel for medical meetings or pleasure, to forget the carnage for a day or two. The trips afforded solace and an opportunity to recharge our emotions. None of us had utilized our official R&R, but regional travel afforded welcome relief, as the following day proved.

I flew to Can Tho for a meeting of delta MILPHAP teams. Before the first lecture, I chatted with Dr. John O'Malley, a plastic surgeon from Orlando who was visiting the delta after two months as an AMA volunteer in Da Nang. He described atrocities inflicted on captured children of ARVN soldiers. The kids were subjected to a barbaric procedure. VC placed blasting caps in the children's mouths, then detonated them—with unspeakable results. O'Malley told me operating on the young victims was the most painful experience of his career.

The meetings commenced on a more pleasant note—medical care for Chieu Hoi (repatriation program) "open arms" returnees. More than 30,000 of these former VC had surrendered within the past year and the program was hailed as a cost-effective success. To kill one VC by military action was estimated to cost $40,000, but to repatriate a Chieu Hoi, a mere $160. If the statistics were correct, the program was certainly effective. Repatriation produced many refugees, together with their families, but life in repatriation centers was harsh. The speaker outlined efforts to improve their lot, as I recalled Bac Lieu's wretched Chieu Hoi site.

A subsequent discussion was less optimistic and confirmed my suspicion not all MILPHAP teams enjoyed the full support of their medicine chief. The speaker described friction with some chiefs with poor cooperation, hostility, and inefficiency. Few were as well trained or dedicated as Dr. Vinh, and some actively or passively resisted the teams' efforts. As I listened, I felt reassured to work with Vinh.

As a pleasant climax to the meeting, the MILPHAP doctors were flown to Con Son Island for an afternoon of relaxation. A C-47 provided transport to the South China Sea haven 40 miles offshore. Flying over the coast we viewed mud flats, which extended far into the ocean, blending the brown shoreline with the deep blue of the ocean's shelf.

It was a short walk from the runway to a white sandy beach. The island is a tropical paradise, with thick jungles, blue-topped mountains, palm trees, waterfalls, and lush pools that empty into the ocean. Wild orchids thrive in the jungle, which is home to many gaily colored birds. Offshore are coral reefs and an abundance of sea life. As we strolled the beach, fishermen cast their nets into the surf, yielding jack crevalle, needle fish, bass, sand sharks, and perch. Nearby the hulk of a 90-foot fishing trawler was lying on its beam ends on the sand. Several doctors climbed aboard the rusting boat for pictures.

The island had been a prison compound and a penal colony since the days of the French. In 1967, it housed approximately 4,000 political and civilian prisoners, plus 2,000 residents. Several inmates were on the beach, selling hand-made curios as we ate our picnic lunch. I briefly traded beers with friendly Australian physicians but couldn't compete with their drinking skills. Some swam in the gentle surf.

Con Son, also known as Con Dao, is the largest island of the Con Dao archipelago off the southern coast of VN in the South China Sea. During the war it contained the infamous "Tiger Cages" in which prisoners were held under poor conditions. The prison was closed in 1975 and the island is now a tourist attraction featuring luxury hotels.

After an afternoon on the island, we returned to Can Tho and I hitched a ride to Bac Lieu to attend Vinh's farewell party for Dr. Passafaro.

The next morning, I was again airborne, as Don and I accompanied Dr. Passafaro to Saigon for MILPHAP business. We later met at the Continental Palace hotel for drinks where we saw Dick Swanson of *Life* magazine at the bar. Dick had been in the north covering the war. He told me photographing the fighting in I Corps was less pleasant than documenting Bill Owen. The military action was intense, vivid, and highly lethal.

Chapter Sources

Layne O. Gentry, Kenneth W. Hedlund, Ralph F. Wells, et al. "Bacterial Diarrheal Diseases." Chapter 16 in *Internal Medicine in Vietnam, Vol. II: General Medicine and Infectious Diseases.* Edited by Andre J. Ognibene and O'Neill Barrett, Jr., Washington, D.C.: U.S. Government Printing Office, 1982.

Marcia B. Goldberg and Robert H. Rubin. "The Spectrum of Salmonella Infection." *Infectious Disease Clinics of North America* 2, no. 3 (1988): 571–98.

Lloyd G. Stevenson. "Exemplary Disease: The Typhoid Pattern." *Journal of the History of Medicine and Allied Sciences* 37, no. 2 (1982): 159–81.

J. B. Thompson. "Typhoid Fever in Medical History." *Journal of the Tennessee Medical Association* 67, no. 12 (1972): 991–97.

Louis Weinstein. "Tetanus." *New England Journal of Medicine* 289, no. 24 (1974): 1293–6.

R. W. Apple. "Bernard Fall Killed in Vietnam by a Mine While With Marines." *New York Times*, February 21, 1967.

Bernard Fall. *Street Without Joy.* Harrisburg, PA: Stockpole Books, 1961.

Graham Greene. *The Quiet American.* London: William Heinemann, 1955.

8

March

Terror, Birth Control—Bac Lieu Style

I entered my fifth month in Vietnam having witnessed many examples of VC brutality, exceeded by the sheer might of U.S. weaponry. The enemy was ruthless in its application of violence, with atrocities so heinous they were difficult to comprehend. Casualties inflicted by helicopters or ARVN military were equally awesome, with a steady procession of the slaughtered. The devastation was palpable, but I had yet to become a target of the VC's enmity, which would suddenly change. The event affected my emotions for years to come.

At 11:25 p.m. on March 1, I was awakened by two thunderous noises in rapid succession, followed by a hail of debris hitting the roof of our hooch. Incoming rounds!

Don and I scrambled out of our bunks and ran to the bunker immediately behind our hooch as a third blast exploded near the motor pool. I stumbled on the wooden planks, tumbling into a muddy ditch before I made it to the bunker. I cursed a skinned knee as we were joined by two officers from the adjacent hooch. The terrible noises continued for a few minutes, shells landing elsewhere in the compound, others near our hooch. More men entered the bunker, clad in shorts. Some carried helmets, a few managed to bring clothes or a weapon. The next few minutes were the most terrifying of my life. I sat with head between knees, crouched in a corner of the small sandbag enclosure with my comrades. One shell exploded immediately on the other side of sandbags behind which I cowered, causing a loud ringing in my left ear that became a permanent hearing defect.

During a lull in the explosions Don and I ran to our hooch to fetch .30 caliber machine gun ammunition stored below our desk. Approximately five minutes after the attack began, we heard "out-going stuff" by the 105 mm howitzers. The fusillade by the ARVN artillery was intense, but enemy shells continued to fall for several long, agonizing minutes. As the tempo of the attack lessened, Don and I went to our hooch, quickly dressed then ran to the latrine where medical supplies were stored and medical personnel were to rendezvous. Steve, Stoney, Mariana, and Joan were helping two ARVN soldiers with minor injuries. After dressing their wounds, we proceeded to the hospital.

Multiple patients filled the ER. Jim had been at the hospital during a maternity call and was assisting Dr. Vinh in surgery. A policeman who guarded the hospital was lying on the floor, eviscerated. On a nearby exam table a woman with three missing limbs and multiple chest wounds gasped for air and died moments later. Other wounded were scattered throughout the room tended by anxious families. Linda, Pat, and our medics arrived to initiate triage of the most severely injured who were salvable. Those with lesser wounds were relegated to wait. Patients with obviously fatal wounds were placed in a corner and given morphine when it became available. Control of visitors became a priority.

I went to surgery and scrubbed with Vinh on the policeman's injuries. As I stepped into the operating room, I saw Spooky dropping flares and firing tracers. The fixed-wing craft was closely followed by three helicopters that sprayed the scene with machine guns and rockets.

Spooky was the C-47 two-engine cargo plane adapted for night warfare and equipped with multiple guns controlled by the pilot as well as flood lights. The craft was also called "Puff the Magic Dragon."

The pace of new casualties accelerated. Charlie sent some to be fluoroscoped as Don helped corpsmen and the nurses with triage and crowd control. The northern sky was ablaze with explosions and a continuous staccato of red streaked from Spooky and the choppers. Blasts from bombs dropped from fighters sounded very close and shook the ground.

The next major case was a pregnant woman hit in the abdomen with shrapnel. A large metal fragment narrowly missed her six-month gravid uterus but damaged several pelvic blood vessels with considerable bleeding.

As night merged to morning, the parade of the mutilated was unabated—at least 100 had presented to the hospital and we had treated more than 50 patients by 9:00 a.m. People walked, were carried, or arrived in cyclos, taxis, or buses. Hospital and MILPHAP staffs took short breaks. No one accumulated more than an hour or so of rest, and no sleep. Dr. Vinh departed at 8:00 a.m. As he left, he inspected his Land Rover. When he drove to the hospital during the barrage, a shell exploded a few meters from his car. Luckily, he saw no damage to his vehicle and drove home. During a break I walked to our hooch, passing a gaping crater just behind where I had crouched and a fallen tree adjacent to our bunker.

At 10:30 a.m., I returned to the hospital to observe a fresh traffic jam. Now the pedicabs, taxis, and other vehicles drove past the ER to the morgue, where more than 20 bodies were neatly arranged on the cement floor. Some had been placed in plastic sacks, others lay uncovered for identification. Many were children. The charred remains of one victim were piled in a corner.

That afternoon Vinh and the police chief drove us downtown to survey the city's damage. By this time, we knew there were at least 35 dead and more than 100 injured. The search for additional victims in the rubble occupied police and civilians who looked for missing family members.

We saw ARVN bunkers that had sustained direct hits, and homes that were little more than shacks where entire families perished. There were holes in roofs, mud and shrapnel-spattered structures, and pock-marked trees and buildings as well as craters left by exploding rounds. On the MACV compound one shell landed adjacent to the chapel, peppering the building and drilling holes in the brass bell that calls to worship. Amazingly, the new electric organ had not been damaged.

Across the river the ARVN ammunition dump was smoldering. Thousands of rounds of shells, grenades, mortars, and other explosives littered the area, many unspent. The ARVN dependents living near the site suffered the most—a substantial number of the injured and dead came from that locale. An area the size of a block had been leveled by the intense heat and secondary explosions. Among the ruins, one could identify remnants of beds, chairs, and other furniture. A group of soldiers were placing charred bones into bags—the only remains of those caught in the inferno.

Late that afternoon rumors circulated of another VC attack. On hearing the news, the tight feeling in my throat and gut returned.

The rumors were true. At 9:15 p.m., the first round exploded in the compound, destroying the MARS radio station. Everyone ran to their bunkers as the alarm sounded. The next shell hit an EM hooch. The attack was short—perhaps 15 or 20 minutes—but the shelling was intense. It became clear several weapons from different locations were firing simultaneously. The ARVN 105s' response was swift, and gunships were quickly in the air. We rendezvoused at the latrine as before. There were no casualties in the compound, so we ran to the hospital.

In the ER a teenage girl with multiple fragments in her chest awaited me. I rapidly did a cutdown on a vein for IV fluid access and drained her chest of blood, but she died within minutes. Other victims came and went—skull fractures, abdominal wounds, amputations—a myriad of gore. Like the previous night, darkness melted into dawn as work on the victims proceeded.

The VC recoilless rifle crews had good aim. Most of the shells hit the MACV

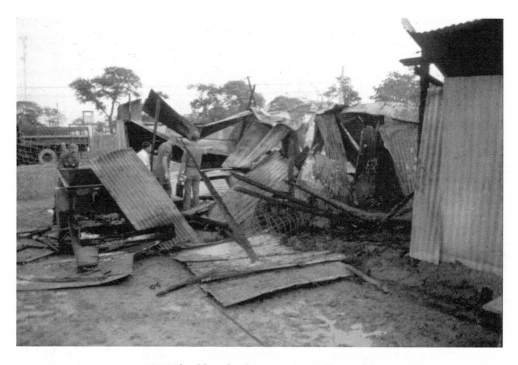

ARVN building hit by 75 mm recoilless rifle.

compound or nearby. Two or three landed on hospital grounds, and one blew out the walls of a ward. Luckily, no patients were present.

A dud landed behind the kitchen and another exploded in front of the hospital. The ARVN medical aid area was hit, inflicting five deaths. Vinh was very agitated when he learned of explosions in the hospital.

The second night's attack by recoilless rifles and mortars led to 12 dead and two dozen injured of those who made it to the hospital. At noon I saw bodies in the morgue in wooden coffins, bedecked in silks and covered with bananas for putrefaction. Don found the head of a recoilless rifle shell embedded in the wall of Ward 4– one could read the Chinese lettering on the grisly souvenir.

The 75 mm recoilless rifle has been utilized by multiple countries since World War II. During the VN war, the VC employed weapons from several sources, including Chinese and those captured from the Americans. The gun is portable and light weight, and can be set up and fired by two individuals, making it a favorite of the VC. It was originally designed as an antitank weapon, although it was an artillery piece in the hands of the VC. A smaller caliber gun was sometimes used, but the 75 mm was the VC's favorite. With reasonable accuracy, it could fire a 20-pound projectile filled with high explosives over a range of 4–5 km.

No enemy had been captured or killed during the attacks, although the firing positions were located. It was estimated a platoon-sized group were involved. More than 80 of the 75 mm shell casings were found at one site of the shooting.

The following day, the VC distributed leaflets in the city proclaiming they would

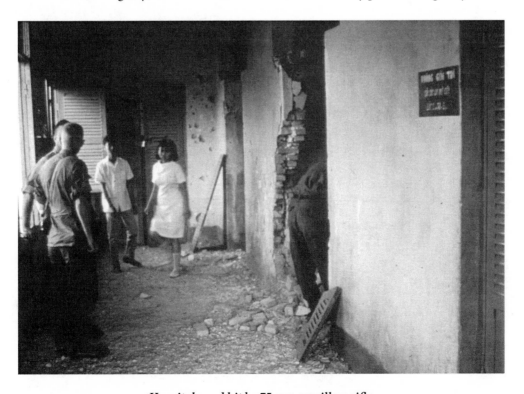

Hospital ward hit by 75 mm recoilless rifle.

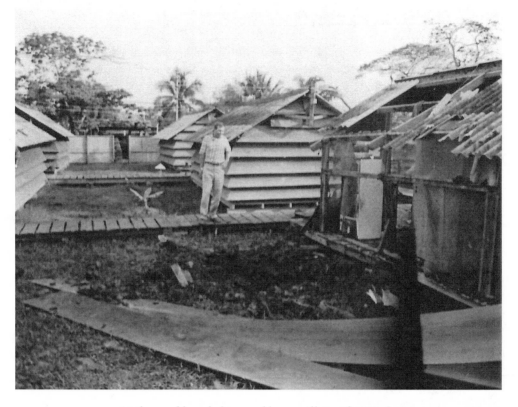

Author and hooch damaged by recoilless rifle attack.

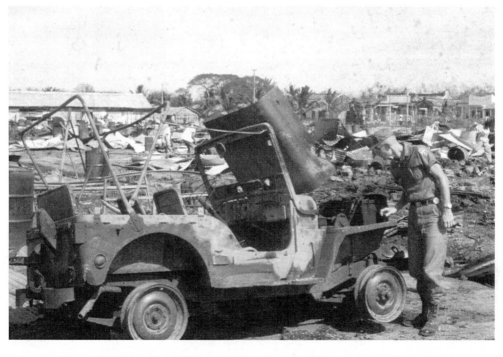

Don Robinson and smoldering ammo dump hit by 75 mm recoilless rifle.

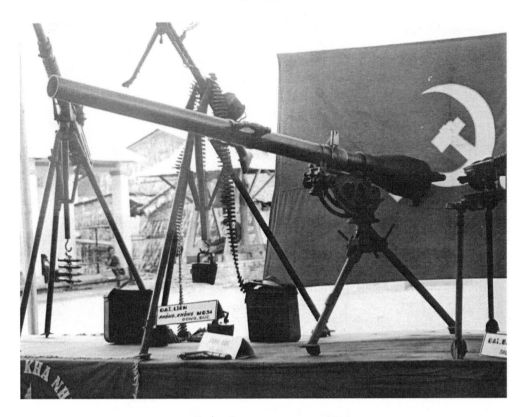

75 mm recoilless rifle among captured VC weapons.

"destroy" Bac Lieu during the next several days. Civilians were frightened and several employees, including hooch girls, asked for money to travel to Soc Trang where it was thought to be safer. Many hospital workers did not report for work and several downtown merchants shuttered their businesses.

An operation was mounted to locate the culprits. Gunships and jets dropped bombs and made rocket runs within earshot. The airfield was alive with choppers carrying troops, nicknamed "slicks," as well as other aircraft.

We made rounds in and around the hospital. People had set up hammocks and mosquito nets, seeking protection along the sides of hospital buildings.

The compound was a scene of intense activity—loading sandbags, stocking reinforcements, repairing bunkers, and receiving supplies. There were rumors of another attack.

The evening was alive with noise and light—gunships patrolled overhead, and the 105 mm artillery bombardment began early. The three-million candle power flare ships and Spooky were aloft throughout the night. The VC did not attack.

Our team met in the morning to assess recent events and update our emergency plans, followed by hurried rounds, which focused on post-op patients. Emergency medications and other items arrived from Can Tho, replenishing those consumed during the attacks. The hospital had treated more than 100 victims in two days, with remarkably favorable results considering our limited capabilities.

We thankfully experienced a quiet night, although there was considerable action nearby. Captain Dan Vento flew in a gunship patrol, and his chopper received heavy automatic weapons fire. Other helicopters were called to assist, and the battle was joined. Gunships returned to base twice to rearm. Despite the amount of armor thrown at them, the enemy continued to shoot at the aircraft.

Night call had become potentially dangerous. When we exited the rear gate to the hospital grounds, the new ARVN guards challenged us. More than once, we startled the nervous recruits in the dark. Before we could identify ourselves, weapons were drawn and directed at us. A fatal accident could result from such an encounter. An armed EM now escorted us on our evening visits to the hospital.

Considering recent events, the Sunday that followed was a normal day and only a few wounded came to the ER: victims of the evening gunship exercise. Our team took the opportunity for some much-needed rest.

That afternoon I treated an old man who was shot by an ARVN guard at a local outpost. The unfortunate man wandered too close to the sentry and received several bullet wounds. He died during surgery.

On Monday we flew to Gia Rai to visit the rural health station. The chopper's flight became more interesting than planned. Gia Rai was situated on one of the main canals 35 km south of Bac Lieu, a disputed zone of control between ARVN and VC, and the origin of considerable conflict. One year earlier the outpost was overrun and all but one U.S. soldier killed. There was intense daily VC activity, and it was thought the recoilless rifle teams resided nearby.

Our chopper came in fast and low, made two passes and landed quickly on the road near the canal. The subsector commander, a major, ran to greet us—obviously upset. Our pilot had been using the wrong radio frequency and couldn't hear the ground transmissions for landing instructions. The major had tried to warn the pilot of an ARVN artillery barrage. We flew directly through the firing of the 105s as we approached, a tragedy narrowly averted among the many "accidents of war." Our visit was uneventful, although the clinic personnel told us they lived in constant fear.

A divisional operation was held near Gia Rai the next day. Light contact was made but several VC prisoners were taken. I hoped the action would provide some relief to those stationed at Gia Rai.

A heavy 105 mm blitz ensued that evening—more than 100 rounds of H&I were volleyed, each round costing more than $100. War is an expensive enterprise.

The morning 'bou brought Dr. William Woodruff, our latest AMA volunteer doctor. A general surgeon, he practiced in Vallejo, California, with the Kaiser group and his weather-beaten face bespoke prior service in the Navy in World War II and Korea. We didn't mention the recent attack and Bill was relieved when told he could rest for the remainder of the day, as he had been in transit several days. After dinner we gave him a tour of the hospital. His discomfort upon viewing the status of the facility was obvious. I was shocked to see faces fall with their first view of the hospital. In the few months since my arrival, I had become inured to our primitive operation.

Dr. Woodruff met the medicine chief the next morning, and the two surgeons assessed one another. Vinh began with his usual question, "What do you think of

Bac Lieu?" Woodruff managed a weak answer: he would need time to form an opinion. He paused for a few moments then startled everyone, especially Dr. Vinh, by asking a question in French. The icebreaker did the trick, and soon the two were chatting in French like old friends. Woodruff had clearly scored a personal victory and Vinh was delighted with his new surgical colleague.

The threat of another attack led to increased defensive action. The artillery began its nightly roar earlier than usual as I walked to Jim's hooch to borrow books from his "lend lease" library. I obtained two novels by Nikos Kazantzakis and a Joseph Conrad volume. Jim was a not only a font of medical knowledge but enriched my taste in literature. Before I departed, he reminded me of his plans for a new maternity program. He gave no details except two words: Planned Parenthood. My curiosity was now fully whetted as he'd been thinking of the project for two months. I had multiple hooch chats with Jim. He was a wise counsel and a major influence of my subsequent career. Jim held liberal views on most topics, which were well supported as he read extensively. He disclosed little of his personal life, but loved to discuss literature, medicine, and especially politics.

Rumors and more rumors—terrorism is one portion threat, one part hostile action and ten helpings of gossip. We learned of heightened security precautions, but one of the VN nurses cheerfully remarked, "All the VC have gone home—we are safe again." During lunch an intelligence officer confirmed several local VC battalions remained active. One could choose to believe whatever story you wished.

We received two patients from the recent Gia Rai operation. One was a young girl with a minor head wound. The note accompanying the patient said her father

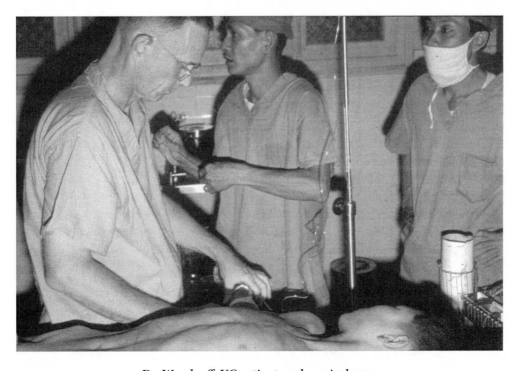

Dr. Woodruff, VC patient, and surgical crew.

had been killed as he and other members of a VC company attempted to overrun an outpost. She was shot by a chopper as she carried ammunition to her father. When I examined her, she was calm but distrustful, and did not resist my actions.

Vinh and Woodruff performed several surgical cases, jabbering away in French as they operated.

The 105s artillery battery now started early in the evening and continued throughout the night, with an occasional charge 7 round, the largest explosive, with the longest range. The bark of the guns shook our hooch and jarred eardrums. Spooky and a light ship were aloft during the hours of darkness.

Three additional patients were evacuated from Gia Rai for surgery. Drs. Woodruff and Vinh had established a bond of friendship and Woodruff was now well adapted to the routine of "Bac Lieu General Hospital."

I made another trip to Gia Rai to discuss the dangerous situation of our health staff and restock items. We returned over salt flats near the sea. The pilot told me they were controlled by VC and the annual salt harvest would exceed hundreds of tons. Money from the sale supported the VC's delta activities and accounted for nearly 25 percent of their budget. To pacify and subsequently occupy the area would require a large body of ARVN troops. In turn, destroying the region with chemical weapons would make it unfit for many years. Thus, the VC ran the nearby salt operation with relative impunity.

We also flew over a VC canal block, a checkpoint to extract tributes. Multiple attempts to destroy the structure had been made, but there were insufficient ARVN troops to complete the mission and occupy the site, like the salt operation. Accordingly, two permanent VC fortifications surrounded by friendly villagers existed within 20 km of Bac Lieu. The salt flats and canal block were two of many oddities in a bizarre war.

The VC attacked USAID facilities in Ca Mau, although their efforts were ill-timed. A bomb was planted at USAID headquarters, but it detonated when no personnel were present. Rumors circulated that Bac Lieu USAID personnel will be targeted. Dr. Woodruff, who bunked with the USAID representative, was not elated by the news.

One of the officers gave me a leaflet the VC had distributed downtown. Co Phung translated the message, which said they vowed to destroy the MACV compound and kill USAID personnel, confirming the earlier rumor. I didn't show the paper to Bill Woodruff.

Intelligence sources identified the locations where recoilless rifles had recently fired on Bac Lieu. Three ARVN battalions were airlifted to a position north of the city, and the oversize cordon of men converged on the suspected sites. A company-sized unit of VC were briefly engaged, but they practiced their usual legerdemain, disappearing into the countryside and eluding capture. No weapons were found. The afternoon sky was alive with planes and slicks returning the unsuccessful troops to base.

Attempts at normalcy were juxtapositioned with war's reality. We had been attacked a few days earlier, and both the city and the MACV compound bore scars of the recent shelling. But life included mundane and pleasant events as welcome respites from the war. The nurses hosted a pizza party at their downtown home. They lived in a large two-story cement structure once owned by a wealthy French merchant. Charlie brought three bottles of Chianti, which we sipped as the pizza baked. After the first batch of pies, the stove's butane supply was exhausted and the second set took longer to cook over a one-burner kerosene stove. Luckily, there was sufficient wine to bridge the gap. The conversation was benign but animated: U.S. national parks, vacations, people's homes, and schools. The girls acknowledged their families feared for their safety, but the elephant in the room, the recent attacks, was not mentioned.

At midnight we were awakened by a terrific explosion just after a 105 mm artillery round had been fired. Some men started for their bunkers, but there were no subsequent blasts. The following morning, we learned one of the 105 mm rounds with a VT (variable timing) fuse exploded immediately after leaving the gun—decapitating one of the weapons crew. VT fuses are delicate devices at the head of the shell, preset to detonate at a specified time after firing. There was an ARVN military funeral in the afternoon.

Over his customary rum and Coke in the officers' club, Bill Woodruff reflected on his status. In his southern drawl he offered, "Hell, this is my third war, but in this one I stand a fair chance of being shot." He spent another operating day with Dr. Vinh, including two casualties and a boy with a harelip. Bill served in both World War II and Korea and was again in harm's way, this time as a volunteer.

Armed Forces News reported renewed VC attacks upon MACV installations, including shelling three units in the Delta. I awoke to artillery fire and the sound of small arms. Two outposts near town were overrun, and Vi Thanh's outpost was attacked. VC crept to the compound's gate and detonated two claymore mines. Col. Wilkins was in the compound and the first blast shook him out of his bunk. Two ARVN soldiers were seriously injured. In the morning Col. Maddox visited one of the outposts. Delta attacks had obviously accelerated, and everyone was on edge, but much greater lethality was occurring to the north in I, II, and III Corps. Military radio reported 232 American deaths and more than 1,300 injured for the week ending March 8. The grim statistic was nearly duplicated March 18, with 211 deaths: four-fold the losses during November.

I was called from the evening movie to treat four policemen hit by grenades tossed at their jeep. Tired and disappointed from the unending stream of injured, I trudged to my hooch where the nightly artillery cannonade nudged me to sleep, although not very gently.

At breakfast Tom Needham clarified some military data. He said the 42nd Divisional Tactical Area (DTA) for the 21st ARVN division represented nearly 20 percent of VN's land mass, an area the size of Louisiana and Mississippi. The DTA was almost as large as III Corps, which housed the greatest concentration of VC. But in III Corps there were 36 battalions of combined American and ARVN troops, predominately American. A U.S. battalion (BTN) is 900–1,000 men. An ARVN BTN averaged 500 personnel. There were nearly as many VC in our DTA, but the 21st ARVN division had only two battalions, plus two ranger battalions and virtually no American troops. Unless the United States substantially increased forces in the delta, the VC would continue to enjoy a healthy superiority. The depressing news roiled my emotions as I walked to the hospital the next morning.

Staff Sergeant James Parker arrived, a new addition to our MILPHAP team, which had risen to 19 members.

Vinh and Woodruff were closing the abdomen of a typhoid surgery when several loud thuds shook the operating room. It wasn't immediately clear if the explosions were incoming. Charlie and I were watching the procedure and ran outside to confirm it was friendly fire. Reassured, the surgeons finished the case, conversing in French.

I would depart the following morning for Can Tho, but that evening Jim invited me to his hooch to unveil his maternity project, a family planning clinic. Disease and malnutrition resulted in high infant and child mortality in rural VN. Vietnamese women were chronically ill and malnourished, but bore many children, as half their offspring would not survive to adulthood. Contraception was virtually unknown in the country, but Jim believed a family planning clinic could achieve smaller, healthier families. He had discussed the project with the chief midwife, and she and her group were enthusiastic. IUDs (intra-uterine devices) were promised by Jim's friends in the United States, and he planned to initiate the "Planned Parenthood" clinic within a few days. I agreed and marveled of his insight.

In Can Tho we were given an update on loss of medical supplies between Saigon and the provinces. John Marsh said USAID was virtually helpless to control the fate of matériel once it was unloaded and became the responsibility of the Ministry of Health (MOH). Theft occurred directly on the docks. Additional disappearance ensued during distribution; one-half or less of a shipment typically arrived at its destination. Marsh said USAID and MACV repeatedly complained to the government, but multiple layers of corruption and mismanagement were beyond their control. Don and I were depressed but not surprised. Marsh urged patience but gave little optimism the situation would improve. It seemed our partners in the war were unable or unwilling to address the rampant graft that sapped our mutual efforts.

These activities were not isolated. Extensive corruption occurred in multiple branches of the government. The duplicity was worse during the Diem regime, but ongoing with the current government, creating fortunes for many Vietnamese officials as it bolstered support for the VC.

The Can Tho meeting concluded with helpful lectures on dengue, malaria, and plague. Malaria remained a major problem in VN, although the disease was less common in the delta than areas with more vegetation. But most cases in VN were due to *Plasmodium falciparum*—the most treacherous form.

Malaria has been a scourge in Vietnam for centuries. Soldiers of the Mongol ruler Kubla Khan of Coleridge's famous poem who were sent to establish a trade route to India became ill. Centuries later, the French battled the infection, particularly in the forests of the central highlands where they cultivated the cinchona tree to extract quinine. The tree is native to Peru, and transplantation to Europe was mistakenly attributed to the Spanish Countess of Chinchon, the woman immortalized in Goya's painting. Hence the tree's name, although an "H" was somehow lost in translation. The bark has been used to treat malaria since the 1600s, although quinine was not extracted until 1820.

American military involvement with malaria in VN was characterized by three problems: rapid development of drug-resistant forms of *Falciparum* malaria; insecticide resistance by the *Anopheles* mosquito; and failure of many soldiers to take the weekly chloroquine-primaquine (CP) prophylaxis. From 1965 through 1970 more than 24,000 cases of malaria were documented in U.S. troops, with 400,000 sick days and more than 40 deaths. Malaria became the most significant U.S. military medical problem, and the *Falciparum* variety accounted for 75 percent of illness, quickly becoming resistant to primaquine and requiring the need for multidrug therapy. Although the CP pill was given as prophylaxis, many soldiers didn't take it because of side effects, forgetfulness, or other factors. Nearly 10 percent of Black troops suffered from hereditary G6pD deficiency, which ironically may have evolved as a protective mechanism to malaria in Africa. These individuals were prone to jaundice, anemia, and other reactions to primaquine, another factor that reduced CP compliance by Black soldiers. We saw few cases of malaria in Bac Lieu but obtained blood smears to search for the parasite in patients with unexplained fever.

I caught a ride to Bac Lieu on a De Havilland Otter. The Toronto company produced three aircraft used extensively by the U.S. military in VN—the Otter, Caribou, and Beaver. All were designed for maximum payload with minimum runway requirements. The Caribou was the largest of the trio and featured the distinctive raised tail section into which cargo could be loaded, while the Otter and Beaver were smaller planes designed for passengers; three vehicles in the vast array of aircraft which populated Vietnam's skies.

At dinner I got an earful from Maj. Blair on the recent VC attack at Vi Tranh. He was spending the night at the outpost, which was guarded by a company of RFPF. VC crept to the entrance where guards were sleeping, blew open the gate, and ran into the compound, setting off satchel charges and firing into hooches. Blair grabbed his .30 carbine and headed for the door as a charge exploded, knocking him back into the room. As he picked himself up, he heard small arms fire and feared the worst. But the VC hit and ran. Blair stumbled to the hooch's door with weapon ready, but the VC had departed. Fortunately, no Americans were killed, although several Purple Hearts were awarded for the night's activities. Within a few days the outpost received additional guards and security measures, including much-needed bunkers.

More travel. I left for Saigon on the 'bou for yet another USAID meeting. The flight to Can Tho was swift, but my Saigon connection was delayed. When I arrived in Saigon the day's meeting had concluded, but I met Boyd Mullholand for dinner. Boyd was the MOC of the MILPHAP team in Quang Nhai near the U Minh forest. His team was battling plague—a horrible disease with high mortality, despite prompt antibiotic therapy.

The briefings were held in the Joint U.S. Public Affairs Office auditorium adjacent to the Rex hotel in downtown Saigon. Most attendees were military and the lectures of little interest to me. But one talk on the Revolutionary Development Program (RDP) piqued my curiosity. The State Department and the Saigon government devoted considerable resources to RDP. A team included approximately

60 members assigned to a newly pacified area to establish local democracy. RD was difficult and dangerous work, as VC infrastructure was heavily concentrated in rural hamlets. VC were courageous and tenacious fighters and often held in high esteem. As Dr. Marsh mentioned, corruption at the local level enhanced the VC's efforts. Thus, even if a hamlet had been "liberated" by government forces, it was difficult to instill commitment of the villagers. RD teams attempted to build local administration and security. But success was often transient and RD personnel were frequently assassinated.

The speaker criticized attempts by the government to win local support with gifts and promises. In contrast, he emphasized RD teams achieved greater success by replacing VC leadership and establishing aid programs. Time would tell. Most of the audience, including me, were skeptical. I thought, "We will not win the war by large military operations. The countryside is key—where Saigon's support is limited."

I went to the 17th field hospital to obtain orthopedic instrument and struck up a conversation with Lt. Col. Don Tilson, a MSC officer. We mutually bemoaned Americans' lack of interest in the plight of VN peasants and the war.

"Life in the U.S. is sweet—people can't be bothered about bombs, murder and corruption in a far distant land," Tilson said, adding, "What frightens me is many soldiers are also apathetic. The average GI doesn't understand the war and just wants to go home. Most Americans don't believe we should be here anyway. I'm not very optimistic." After ruminating a few minutes, Tilson and I concluded neither of us would have much impact on the conflict. Like the song: "Que Sera, sera—What will be, will be." Bidding him adieu, I collected my instruments and returned to the USAID compound in a depressed mood.

Subsequent briefings had no application to me, so I returned to Bac Lieu. The trip south was tedious, and I arrived to begin evening call. The first victim was a man whose arm was amputated in a grisly manner by a helicopter machine gun. As we operated, I thought of my conversation with Col. Tilson.

A large ARVN operation was held the following day, yielding 13 VC killed and 100 prisoners, together with a cache of VC guns, grenades, ammunition, and mortars. Helicopters flew protective missions into the night. Tom Needham was aboard one of the gunships and had a narrow escape. They were flying at 3,000 feet when the pilots suddenly couldn't control the chopper. The ship fell several hundred feet before the descent was halted. Tom was sweating bullets, although the pilot and copilot were unfazed. The cause of the mishap was never detected, but similar malfunctions were

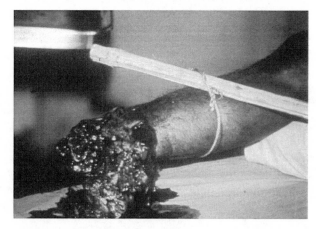

Traumatic amputation by machine gun.

commonplace, and often lethal. War leads to the intersection of complicated and dangerous machinery with variable human input with risk of adverse events—true since war was first conceived by man. War zones are dangerous places.

The next morning Jim initiated the first session of the "Bac Lieu Planned Parenthood" clinic. As OB docs, Jim, Charlie, and I had all seen the effects of primitive abortions and obstetrical complications affecting "multips" (women who have had several pregnancies). Jim placed 15 IUDs, and the turnout was enthusiastic. Several women were turned away as the supply was exhausted. He anticipated receiving additional IUDs within a few days. The midwives were also excited. Jim predicted fewer pregnancies, healthier families, and fewer unwanted pregnancies terminated by abortion, a shady practice in VN and the United States. The *Roe v. Wade* legal battle would be waged in the future and contraception was not widely practiced in America or VN. All abortions were illegal. As an OB trainee I saw the effects of backroom procedures to terminate a pregnancy. The LA County hospital created an infected obstetrics service (IOB) to manage complications of abortions. Residents served rotations on IOB, often admitting more than 30 patients a day suffering from bleeding and infection from incomplete abortions (INCABs). IOB was my introduction to young women dying of septic shock. The busiest time was Monday night, when "Tijuana Specials"

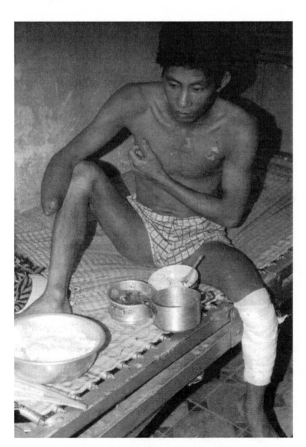

Recovering amputation patient.

would arrive—girls who crossed the border over the weekend to obtain a procedure. I met Barbara Bailey on IOB, where she was head nurse. After a rocky beginning we developed a budding romantic relationship. Although Charlie was Catholic, he had similar experiences during OB training. For the next few months Jim's U.S. colleagues provided a steady supply of IUDs. The approach to contraception was well suited to VN conditions: no requirement for hormone medications, well tolerated, easily reversible, and could be inserted by midwives.

Early one morning one of the psy-war L-19 aircraft buzzed the compound. On its second pass we ran outside to get a look at the intruder. A stern voice boomed from the plane: "Good morning Bac Lieu! Good morning Bac Lieu!" I had yet to identify the prankster, but suspected Maj. McKenna. The plane's loudspeakers were usually employed to entice repatriation of VC for the Chieu Hoi program.

The U.S. news agencies reported the Guam peace conference had concluded, reaffirming strong American support for the Saigon government and no major policy changes. I found it interesting an ambassador named Lodge would be replaced by a Bunker. I chuckled, "That's just what we need in VN—more Bunkers!"

The March 1967 Guam conference included President Johnson, Secretary McNamara, and other senior U.S. personnel, plus Thieu and Ky. Henry Cabot Lodge Jr., U.S. ambassador from 1965, was replaced by Ellsworth Bunker, a hardline supporter of American involvement. U.S. commitment to South Vietnam was strengthened with plans to expand military forces and increased funding.

Tom Needham, our Green Beret local representative, conducted an evening therapy session, or "Doctors' Briefing," which became a frequent diversion. We would assemble in Tom's hooch to receive a tactical and psychological summary of the war with comical overtones. Both ARVN and VC were targets of his lampoons—Tom provided an amusing story to match. The U.S. Army's history of SNAFUs was rich, but combining U.S. advisors with ARVN soldiers multiplied the number and severity of mistakes. In turn, the VC "screwed up" just as often. He presented anecdotes in a humorous, good-natured manner. We all experienced anxiety and difficulty sleeping since the recent attack, so Tom's satires were good medicine. Unfortunately, the humor was quickly dulled as we emerged from his hooch to endure another evening of barrage by the 105s. ARVN outpost positions were plotted by the gunnery crews. If an outpost was attacked, the gunners would put a protective ring of fire within 50 yards of the facility. But the noise fractured attempts of sleep.

Sunday March 26: Easter Sunday: Although it was Easter Sunday, the daily routine was little affected. Following morning services, the chaplain and Catholic priest departed for their tour of outposts. On this day they had a choir, including a USAID nurse, Don Robinson, Capt. Reed, and five MILPHAP enlisted men.

Dr. Woodruff took the holiday to accompany Col. Maddox's visits to ARVN outposts. Near Vinh Long they encountered a heavy battle; five choppers were shot down, killing one pilot. Another pilot and the command chopper, flown by the divisional commander, Col. Dempsey, was hit, killing the colonel. In regions where U.S. forces fought, enlisted men constituted the most casualties. For MACV advisory units, ARVN soldiers suffered the greatest injuries. But if an American was hurt or killed, it was often an officer. As there were only a hundred MACV personnel in Bac Lieu, a death was akin to losing a member of one's family.

By late morning Drs. Vinh and Jones had completed two surgeries plus maternity clinic. Vinh offered to take us on an afternoon excursion. At 1:00 p.m., Dr. and Mrs. Vinh collected the MILPHAP docs for a picnic. Mrs. Vinh looked like a typical American housewife embarking on a weekend outing, with stretch pants, flowered print blouse, sunglasses, and toddler in arms. We drove to a series of Buddhist burial tombs where four or five vehicles were parked. The police chief was standing by a jeep, sipping cognac. As we walked to the picnic, I saw several young men in police uniform or civilian attire carrying M1 carbines or submachine guns. The chief carried his security with him.

The party was well underway when we arrived. A large meal was laid out—salad, egg rolls, chicken, duck, turtle, sausages, watermelon, cheeses, bananas and, of course, cognac. After lunch we toured the Cambodian temples, surrounded by coconut palms and flame trees resplendent with red blossoms. We saw multiple Buddhist shrines. A group of young monks in yellow robes greeted us and we viewed a 15-foot Buddha in one of the temples. Dr. Vinh told us the Buddha's eyes were said to contain diamonds—but covered by paint to deter theft. We snapped pictures and inspected the monks' meager living quarters. Our armed escort followed at close range. Although our VN hosts were Buddhists, they acted more like tourists than fellow worshipers.

The actor James Garner visited Bac Lieu, mingling and dining with officers. He was easygoing and expressed interest in officers' comments, although did not share any personal views of the war. I had concluded celebrities were briefed on appropriate topics for discussion, a fact later subsequently revealed by another visitor.

Sergeants Parker and Klick travelled with me to Gia Rai for a progress report from Spc. Scott. As we flew, the slick's door gunners seemed especially alert. We later learned a VC unit with a .50 cal machine gun had been shooting at choppers in the area. Luckily there was no ground fire and we landed without incident. The district health worker in Gia Rai returned with us to obtain more supplies. He transported equipment by chopper, as items shipped by land would be confiscated by the VC.

Dr. John Marsh brought two officials of the Colombo Plan to Bac Lieu. The Plan is a multinational organization founded in 1950 to support economic and social activities in the Asia-Pacific region. Canada was a major humanitarian participant during the war, although remained neutral. The name reflects its headquarters in Colombo, Sri Lanka.

As part of Canada's assistance, it donated supplies to equip a 200-bed hospital. John and the officials affirmed these items would be distributed to province facilities, including Bac Lieu. We pored over lists of autoclaves, anesthetic apparatuses, beds, blankets, medicines, and other items, which would arrive within a few weeks. It was like Christmas shopping by mail.

In the afternoon Mariana, Joan, and I drove to the Catholic orphanage. There had been little medical aid to the nuns since the onset of Dr. Tot's pregnancy. The orphanage was home to more than 200 children, although those most in need were the 50 or so infants. The plight of these tiny charges was particularly sad. Some were abandoned on the orphanage grounds, others given to the nuns by poor families. Many were the result of VC attacks that killed or displaced parents. Each time I visited the orphanage I was overwhelmed. The nuns dealt with a human catastrophe. Infant mortality exceeded 20–25 percent each month, from malnutrition, diarrheal disease, pneumonia, or other diseases. Mariana furnished clothes and other items donated by friends and relatives in Elmhurst, Illinois.

A vigorous nighttime counterattack by U.S. airpower matched an earlier battle by the VC whose machine guns had been menacing choppers patrolling the region. Americans retaliated with massive force. The helicopters made their usual rounds but circling nearby was Spooky and two Skyraider fighters carrying 500-pound bombs. When the helicopters began drawing fire, a FAC aircraft flown by a captain

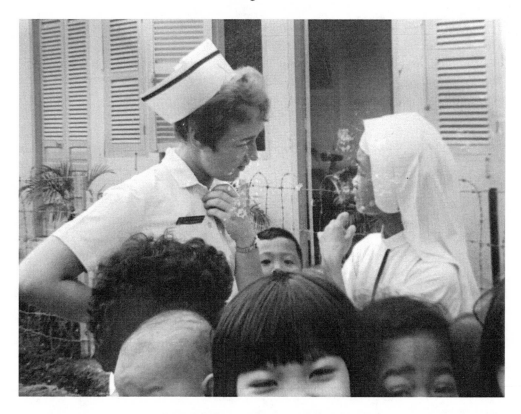

Joan Schubert and nun at orphanage.

identified the enemy locations and called the Skyraiders and Spooky. Although the action occurred several kilometers from the compound, the explosions shook us like a series of earthquakes. The bombs were expended and Spooky followed with its deadly ordnance. I was in the maternity ward and we could see the flares and the bomb bursts. The midwives thought we were under attack, but I said, "Maybay [airplane]," and made mock bomb runs at the floor with my hands. The ward was alive with excitement as we heard the dull, dud-dud-dud of Spooky's mini-cannons.

The Douglas A-l Skyraider was a post–World War II propeller-driven fighter aircraft that carried bombs, torpedoes, and a mini-cannon. The aircraft had a long career after the Vietnam War. An aircraft with a similar name, the Skyhawk, was a jet fighter used extensively in Vietnam.

Late that night I was

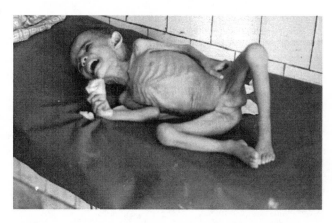

Malnourished orphanage baby (photograph R. Brittis, MD).

called for a VC wounded during the air attack earlier that day. I summoned Dr. Vinh. The victim had multiple lesions and we operated for several hours. The man remained in critical condition. I couldn't imagine the terror inflicted by Spooky and the Skyraiders.

The following morning Don and Pat departed for R&R vacations—Don to Hawaii to meet his wife and Pat to Hong Kong. At 4:00 p.m., I received a call from Don in Saigon, who disclosed their harrowing trip. They flew in an Air America Pilatus Porter. South of Saigon they experienced engine trouble and the pilot radioed for an emergency landing. They set down in a rice paddy, shearing off the wheels as they bounced along the paddy. The landing gear was severely damaged, but the airframe was intact. Almost immediately they received small arms fire from nearby trees. There were only three weapons aboard, but the occupants crawled out and began shooting. Minutes passed and everyone feared disaster. Miraculously, a plane appeared overhead, which fired rockets at the trees. Soon a giant Chinook helicopter landed nearby. The passengers ran to the big chopper and scrambled aboard. The Chinook crew rigged a sling over the bullet-riddled Porter, and within minutes pilot, passengers, and plane were lifted to safety. They landed at Tan Son Nhut, safe, but shaken. What a beginning for an R&R! Don said another Air America plane crashed upcountry, killing all nine passengers. The prospect of a crash is frightening enough—but to then be ambushed is difficult to comprehend.

Two poisonous snakes, a krait and a bamboo viper, were caught in front of Ward 9. I vowed to no longer wear my "kloppers" on evening visits to the hospital.

After clinic I drove Mariana to the Chieu Hoi center for a goodwill trip. She had several bundles of donated clothes. Mr. Zapata, the Chieu Hoi supervisor, helped distribute the gifts to the assembled crowd. Women scrambled to obtain the items as they cradled their babies. It was a scene akin to a bargain basement event.

Jim and Bill Woodruff took the 'bou for a weekend of rest at Vung Tau. Intelligence reported the VC might attack. In anticipation, artillery began its nightly bombardment earlier than normal as an ARVN patrol stumbled onto several VC setting up a 75 mm recoilless rifle. The coordinates were noted and the howitzers blasted away as gunships were dispatched. The attack had been thwarted, but the VC escaped unscathed into the night with their weapon. Because of the excitement, the compound's residents were awake most of the night. I lost sleep for another reason. Two patients added to the growing list of attempted suicides. Victims would take anything—liquid DDT, chloroquine tablets, phenobarbital, folk remedies, or whatever was available. Both patients were teenagers and the ingestions benign. These incidents were stupid but provided relief from the injuries of war and serious infections.

Chapter Sources

O'Neill Barrett, Jr., and Raymond W. Blohm. "Malaria: The Clinical Disease." Chapter 13 in *Internal Medicine in Vietnam, Vol. II: General Medicine and Infectious Diseases*. Edited by Andre J. Ognibene and O'Neill Barrett, Jr., Washington, D.C.: U.S. Government Printing Office, 1982.

Christine Beadle and Stephen L. Hoffman. "History of Malaria in the United States Naval Forces at War: World War I Through the Vietnam Conflict." *Clinical Infectious Diseases* 16, no. 2 (1993): 320–9.

William B. Cohen. "Malaria and French Imperialism." *Journal of African History* 24, no. 1 (1983): 23–36.

Annick Guénel. "Malaria Control, Land Occupation and Scientific Developments in Vietnam in the XXth Century." HAL-SHS 00137031. 1998. Assessed July 2, 2021. https://halshs.archives-ouvertes.fr/halshs-00137031/.

9

April

Trash, Tokyo, and Hepatitis

My sixth month in Vietnam began as usual, on call. We shared the task among MILPHAP and volunteer physicians, with no respite from duty the following day. The first morning of April, I was recalled to the ER after a night on duty and more trauma. The VC planted a booby trap in a nearby hamlet. The blast amputated the right arm of a 12-year-old girl and destroyed her brother's right eye. Their older sister lost both hands, and the father was killed. Vinh and I operated, which delayed our meeting with the Red Cross regarding refugees. Vinh was pleased senior officials took interest in our problems, which were minor compared to Saigon and the northern provinces. Hundreds of thousands of citizens had been uprooted by the war. Many hamlets were abandoned, and people fled to sites near American bases or Saigon for relative safety, creating primitive shantytowns and terrible living conditions. Refugees couldn't find employment and faced hostility from local citizens. A center had been established in Bac Lieu but had little funding. Its tiny staff were unable to process those who arrived every day. Housing conditions were terrible, and food was meager. Vinh drove the officials to the center and introduced them to the staff, although he was not optimistic of remedy. Bac Lieu's refugees endured terrible conditions, but their numbers were few, as many hamlet residents were VC or VC sympathizers, explaining why ARVN operations typically netted few prisoners. The fighters could blend into the countryside, resuming their status as farmers. Vinh presented his views to the officials and dejectedly returned to the hospital—another unresolved dilemma.

Humanitarian disasters involved more than refugees. At lunch Mr. Vick, USAID representative, briefed me on other fiascos of intended goodwill. The U.S. donated many products to Vietnam, including huge amounts of bulgur wheat for distribution to the public. But no one told USAID that Vietnamese cultural mores disfavored bulgur. Thus, tons of grain rotted on Saigon's wharfs or were eaten by rats. Some wheat was ultimately distributed, but villagers either sold it or fed it to hogs. Powdered milk shared a similar problem. Saigon warehouses were bursting with milk, which was also disdained by most citizens, although orphanages, maternity services, and hospitals utilized the product. I was flabbergasted, but Vick was philosophic, explaining the lessons illustrated a mix of supply, needs, and social preference, coupled with cultural ignorance. I shook my head, what a waste.

Charlie witnessed a medical contradiction. He admitted a boy with tetanus whose parents had taken him to a Chinese medicine man because of fever and
cough. The practitioner exorcised the evil spirits with suction cups and incisions
over the child's chest and abdomen. A few days later the boy developed symptoms
of tetanus, which Charlie believed were due to the charlatan's unsterile lacerations.

Another blistering day—the thermometer registered 115 degrees at noon. To
make matters worse, hospital supplies were low, and we were out of aspirin. Three
more suicide attempts presented to the ER, including a boy who drank an insecticide. Despite our efforts, he succumbed that evening. Why did we see so many suicides? The reasons were ludicrous: "She was mad at her boyfriend." Or: "He didn't
like his mother today." The victim's mother followed us throughout the afternoon,
wailing and beating her chest. Her suffering became more tragic as neighborhood
children surrounded her, laughing and taunting. No parents or hospital personnel
intervened, and we ultimately chased away the children. What a land of contrasts.

Each evening now featured intensive 105 mm artillery shelling. More than 7,000
rounds of the howitzers were fired during March, and April was poised to exceed
that number. Sleep, even when not on call, was problematic.

The local repatriation program was relatively successful and many Chieu Hois
surrendered to authorities. But winning a guerrilla war was difficult and slow. A
MACV intelligence officer suggested successful guerrilla warfare required two elements: A weak or corrupt central government and outside aid for insurgents. VN
had both. Massive government graft was coupled with strong rural VC support.
Could Saigon and the United States overcome these obstacles? I was growing progressively skeptical.

U.S. news reported further grim statistics of American losses with more than
1,200 deaths the first three months of 1967. One reason for more accurate casualty fig-
ures may have been eroding public support with demand for transparency. Another
was to refute VC claims of horrendous U.S. losses. Co Anh told me the morning VC
radio broadcast proclaimed 300 Americans were killed in the recent Bac Lieu shell-
ings. We knew no Americans were injured or killed, and the total number of Americans in Bac Lieu was less than 300. But VC propaganda was powerful.

I saw two more suicide attempts as clinics ran at full pace, including 50 kids in
the pediatric clinic. Jim and Bill Woodruff returned from their seaside holiday, tired
and sunburnt. They bought a TV set for Dr. Vinh at the PX and lugged it to Bac Lieu
on the 'bou.

Despite the rash of suicide attempts, war wounds, elective surgeries, and medical crises competed for our attention. After three long procedures Dr. Vinh took off
his mask and lit a Ruby Queen. He remained the unfazed surgeon—grace under fire,
rarely showing emotion, but dedicated to his patients. His stamina was only surpassed by his equanimity.

As Vinh puffed on his cigarette, I raised a topic that had concerned us for several weeks—the hospital incinerator. A nonfunctional stone device sat in a bog
behind the hospital, and we were forced to use 55-gallon drums and kerosene to
burn hospital trash. Children rummaged for discarded bandages, needles, and other
items that escaped the fire. I suggested we build an inclined plane incinerator using

gasoline, from a design Don saw in an Army manual. Vinh liked the plan, but said gasoline was "mac qua"—too expensive. "We don't need gas," he added, "The best fuel is trau." He walked me to the hospital kitchen where "trau," or rice husks, heated the ovens. Rice was abundant, and a large bag of husks cost a few piastres. The husks burnt to a fine ash, which could be discarded or used as fertilizer. Problem solved!

More dog day weather—the thermometer reached 108 as I typed outside my hooch. Dr. Woodruff practiced French on a nearby chaise lounge.

Sgt. Jim Parker and Linda accompanied the hospital team to a school for cholera and smallpox immunizations. Jim attempted to instruct VN staff in the use of the immunization gun, but they required constant supervision and their technique was terrible. For cholera they filled a 5 ml syringe with vaccine, then gave 1 ml doses to five individuals—using the same syringe and needle!

More violence arrived from Gia Rai—three victims with grenade wounds. One boy lost his left hand and part of the right. The victims competed with patients with pneumonia, tetanus, and cholera. At dawn we received three more casualties from Gia Rai who had been shot by an aircraft machine gun, an endless array of crises, all women and children. Gia Rai was our carnage capital. The EMs had devised colorful nicknames for the town—"Gee a Riot," "GR," or simply, "Grrrrr," as a menacing growl.

One morning Vinh and I flew to a local maternity station for an update. On our return he pointed to the small hamlet of Cay Giang, his birthplace. I thought he was from the north, as he attended school and worked in Hanoi for many years. He mentioned his meager beginnings as we flew above Giang's few houses and huts. I asked

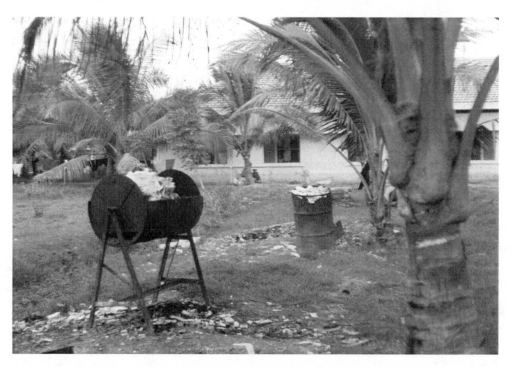

Hospital trash.

about his subsequent education and rise to medical and political prestige, but he waved me off with the promise, "Perhaps another time."

Charlie and I brought medicines to the Catholic orphanage and observed how nuns fed the infants. The process was like the pediatric ward—but worse. The head nun told us they were very frugal with milk, a gross understatement. To provide enough liquid for each child, the nuns added two or three teaspoons of powdered or condensed milk to a cup of water. USAID nurses had instructed the nuns on preparation of milk, but the nuns shunned their efforts or were afraid to exhaust their supply. Most babies had scabies, mosquito bites, open sores, and other rashes, complicated by pneumonia and diarrhea. Despite great handicaps, the nuns saved some lives, but mortality rate was horrendous. Although especially bad in the orphanage, malnutrition was widespread in rural Bac Lieu.

I took a chopper to Soc Trang to see the dentist. On a phone call to Bac Lieu, I learned two boys were admitted with white phosphorus burns from aircraft rockets. The injuries were very severe, and Jim sustained burns as he treated the wounds. The boys were not expected to survive. They were the first but not the last phosphorus victims in Bac Lieu.

After dental work I tried to hitch a ride to Bac Lieu but was unsuccessful, although the delay yielded a bonus. I spent a restful night with no 105s to disturb my sleep.

The morning 'bou was on schedule and I returned to witness the deaths of the boys with phosphorus burns. What an unspeakable weapon.

The days were hot with considerable humidity. I thought the rains might provide a blessing, although they would be accompanied by mud, wet clothes, and mildew. The Vietnamese have a saying: "When the red blossoms fall from the cay diep tree [also called the flame tree], it signals the rainy season." The tree is the official plant of Vietnam.

Jim expanded the "loop" clinic, which had grown rapidly as Jim's stateside friends provided more IUDs. The midwives were eager to participate, but laws of contraception in VN were strict and we proceeded cautiously. Ministry officials soon learned of the project, which led to an ongoing battle to maintain the clinic.

The earth shook as we ate dinner—several air strikes with large bombs were dropped nearby. Casualties were coming.

An ARVN operation yielded many dead and wounded. As allied forces traversed a small canal, they were targeted by automatic weapons and mortar fire. Paratroopers were called to flank the enemy but were outmaneuvered by superior VC forces that pinned down the ARVN troops. One adviser told Steve he'd never seen so many automatic weapons firing at once. In return, VC positions were peppered with machine guns plus mortars. Twenty-four air strikes were called, involving at least 60 aircraft. One Skyraider was shot down. At the end of the fight, the VC body count exceeded 200, with 70 ARVN killed and 170 injured. Many wounded soldiers awaited medical evacuation that evening as troops remained in the field patrolled by Spooky and lightning bugs. The surrounded VC achieved a breakout and the main force escaped into the night, an oft-told tale.

The bloody ARVN battle was followed by further military action. As most VC escaped, a mop-up operation was mounted to search for killed or wounded, as well as destroy bunkers and seize caches of arms. But the VC were resourceful, evacuating as many wounded as possible and hiding their dead. Steve saw several bloodied canal banks where bodies weighted with rocks had been thrown into the muddy water. Others reposed in hastily dug shallow graves.

Estimates of civilians and combatants wounded and killed during the VN conflict are controversial, and the human cost of the war has been difficult to quantitate. Statistics by the Vietnamese MOH and the United States are incomplete, and virtually no data exists for VC killed and wounded. The United States kept accurate records of American injuries and deaths, with more than 47,000 killed in action despite the best medical care. Another 10,000 died of other causes including illness and accidents. In his comprehensive study *America in Vietnam*, Guenter Lewy attempted to quantitate civilian and VN military casualties as well as who inflicted the deaths. Lewy utilized data from provincial hospitals such as Bac Lieu, where monthly results were transmitted to the MOH. Lewy also tabulated the number of civilians admitted to American facilities.

Lewy calculated a minimum of 300,000 civilian deaths from 1965 to 1974. But who was responsible? The question is not easy to answer. Some historians have concluded as many as 80 percent of deaths were directly due to American and ARVN military action. We treated injured civilians after ARVN operations or from bombings and gunships, but believed as many casualties were inflicted by the VC. At least 38,000 civilians were assassinated. To this must be added another 60,000 killed by the VC or NVN. Finally, how many VC and NVN were killed during the conflict? Body counts during operations were notoriously inaccurate. As Steve observed, the VC were innovative in burying, submerging, and otherwise hiding their dead. The number of VC or innocent bystander deaths is therefore an unanswered question. The VN government reported approximately 220,000 soldiers killed, but VC and NVN lives consumed during the conflict may have exceeded 600,000.

Senator Ted Kennedy chaired a U.S. Senate committee to address this issue, using MOH and U.S. hospital data, which suggested at least 475,000 civilian war casualties, substantially more than Lewy's estimates. Others have placed noncombatant losses greater than 600,000, with more than one million civilian deaths over the decades of conflict: ten to twenty-fold the loss of U.S. troops. Those directly killed in the field were also subject to recording errors. Many who died in contested areas were counted as Viet Cong. As Lewy asked, "How can you determine whether black-clad corpses ... were VC or innocent civilians?" For those admitted to hospitals like Bac Lieu, we only knew of deaths in the hospital. VN tradition held if one is not buried by his family, his soul is lost. Severely injured patients were frequently taken from the wards by families to die at home, so hospital statistics tell only part of the story. To compound the tragedy, more than 50 percent of women and children accounted for civilian casualties. This drama unfolded in an underdeveloped country of 16 million engulfed in war for more than two decades. To these numbers must be added hundreds of thousands civilian deaths from disease and malnutrition. Vietnam was severely wounded.

The ARVN military operation proved costly for both sides. In addition to dead and injured, weapons of war are expensive. Nearly 100,000 gallons of fuel were consumed during the two days of fighting involving 70 helicopters, plus food, ammunition, and other supplies for four ARVN battalions. But these costs were minor compared to U.S. operations in I or II Corps, where large-scale army and marine battles raged daily.

The fighting occurred near the U Minh forest, a major VC staging area. A swampy area filled with mangrove trees gave the U Minh its name: "Black Forest." In the past, crocodiles, caimans, and turtles were hunted in the region. The current inhabitants were also clad in black.

On the second day of battle, Steve flew a dust off medevac mission that became a nightmare. The fighting had ceased and the VC broke contact. Steve was flown to examine and evacuate wounded. His chopper and four other ships left the command post for a rendezvous in the forest. The region was a wasteland—ground cover had been burned and the area obscured by thick smoke from rockets and other incendiaries. There were dozens of craters from 500-pound bombs. His ship descended to land, but as they approached the ground, they could see nothing. Where were the wounded? But a score of bedraggled men appeared through the smoke and haze, limping, dragging, or carrying their comrades toward the chopper. The rotors continued to turn, sending up burnt grass, dust, and leaves, making visibility nearly impossible. Many wounded were pulled aboard, and Steve's chopper tried to become airborne as other ships received additional men.

There were too many to be accommodated. Injured soldiers clung to the skids of the last helicopter and the overloaded craft couldn't take off. Crewmen forcibly

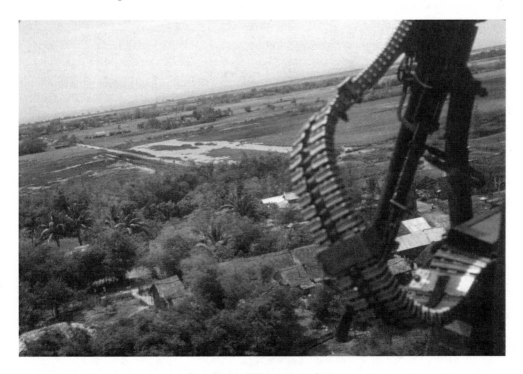

Gunship at VC-contested site.

ejected several injured men, allowing the chopper to achieve flight. Suddenly, Steve heard several sharp cracks and the door gunner yelled, "We're taking fire!" as he readied his machine gun. The ship gained altitude, but tracers arced toward them from a tree line. They were soon out of range and all ships arrived safely at the command post.

Steve witnessed more action as he returned to Bac Lieu in the command chopper with Gen. Minh and Col. Maddox. Near the city, the pilot handed the headset to Col. Maddox, who quickly gave it to the general. The pilot was ordered to alter course. A ranger patrol had come upon a company-sized unit of VC hiding in huts along a canal. After radio transmission with the ground unit, the command chopper made several passes over the huts as the door gunners fired their machine guns. Additional choppers joined the attack with rockets and machine guns.

At 11:00 p.m., I was called to the ER for a 12-year-old boy who had been shot by a "maybay" (aircraft). Both parents and a grandparent had been killed. I called Dr. Vinh and within minutes we were in the operating room. We removed a 7.62 mm bullet from the posterior wall of the boy's stomach, the caliber of a Huey's machine guns. The boy had been in one of the huts Steve described from the command chopper. His family were probably VC. Alternatively, they could have been innocent bystanders, as VC used civilians as shields and sought refuge in their homes. If this were the case, the family's casualties were collateral damage. In a guerrilla war, indigenous people suffered the most, whether innocent or insurgents. Who was responsible for the deaths—the Americans or the VC? This dilemma was a microcosm of civilian casualties throughout the country.

The war was a panoply of many contradictions—those who fought the hardest were our enemy. They were also the most dedicated and could rightfully be called patriots who inspired thousands of peasants to haul weapons, food, and equipment to Dien Bien Phu, enabling Gen. Giap to defeat the French in 1954. The determination of the Viet Minh and their successors made them the best guerrilla fighters in the world. Although the VC inflicted tremendous suffering, the United States was not innocent. The weapons we employed were awesome: Spooky, B-52s, phosphorus, napalm, and much more.

A different story awaited Charlie in clinic. He examined a young child whose mother had taken the boy to a "VC doctor." Folk medicines were given, as well as antibiotics, but the child did not improve. Several days passed. Finally, as related by the interpreter, the VC medic threw up his hands in exasperation, telling the mother to go the "hoa ky" bac si (American doctor).

Charlie wrote regularly to his new wife and his large Italian American family, who reciprocated with an unending series of parcels of wine, salami, and other goodies. Occasionally, a bottle would be broken in shipment, leading to a red-stained package in the mail room, but most parcels arrived in good condition. Charlie was anxious to return to the States, his wife, and complete training, but didn't disclose many personal details. He and Jim shared a hooch and Charlie was often the third member of our evening discussions. His political views were more conservative than Jim's or mine, but we had no serious disagreements.

The next day initiated my R&R in Tokyo. All military personnel were entitled to

R&R (Rest and Recuperation). One could select an in-country site such as Vung Tau (army) or Da Nang (marine), as well as several countries in Asia or Hawaii. Some destinations required a specified length of service or were restricted to officers. The duration of R&R was listed as five days, but with travel, soldiers were typically absent at least a week. Application for R&R was a formal process and travel required orders.

I selected Tokyo and wrote Barbara Bailey to share my holiday. It was a big request—asking a young single girl to fly alone several thousand miles to another country for a tryst. I was delighted when I received her letter of acceptance.

On my flight from Saigon, I read a *Time* magazine, which gave details of the war's escalation and rising opposition in the United States. One article described Martin Luther King's fiery denouncement of U.S. involvement in a landmark speech as massive antiwar demonstrations were held across the country. Muhammad Ali refused military service and was stripped of his boxing title. But protests did not deter the military. Several large marine and army operations were initiated in April. I was happy to have a hiatus from the conflict as I neared Japan.

My flight was on time, but I was delayed several hours at the air base. Barbara was alone in a strange Tokyo hotel. I couldn't contact her, and she didn't know if or when I would arrive. At 1:30 a.m., I finally knocked on her door, and we had a lovely, romantic reunion. The eve of my departure to VN we had enjoyed a farewell dinner at a Japanese restaurant overlooking Hollywood. It seemed prophetic our next meeting would be in Tokyo. I had met Barbara at the LA County hospital. After a few cool social encounters, I was encouraged to pursue Barb by a fellow OB resident. Our first date was an afternoon at the tap room of a local brewery. That humble meeting had blossomed into a serious relationship prior to my Vietnam adventure.

We had wonderful, exciting days exploring Japan—the tall, blond girl in the yellow coat, object of attention by Japanese kids. We visited Nikko, dined elegantly at the Tokyo tower, and took several meals at the Tokyo train station where we pointed to plastic food replicas to select our choices. A highlight was a visit to Howard Corning, a Harvard cardiologist I met during training in Texas. He treated us to a traditional Japanese dinner and bath at his rented home in the Tokyo suburbs.

R&R was over too quickly, and I boarded a jet for Vietnam as Barbara returned to Los Angeles. My thoughts were somber as I approached Saigon; a quiet, reflective ride.

It rained, but the monsoon season would not officially begin for another month. The rice paddies were dry and brown as I rode the 'bou to Bac Lieu.

Col. Maddox had departed for his R&R and Gen. Minh was vacationing in Dalat. Accordingly, no major ARVN operations were scheduled. We hoped the VC would honor the unilateral truce, although the howitzers began their nightly blasts at 8:00 p.m., generating the familiar tight feeling in the stomach and poor sleep. Welcome back to VN!

The actor Efrem Zimbalist, Jr., visited on a "handshake" tour and I chatted with him as we shaved. Performers usually spent two weeks in country, visiting troops and giving shows. Their schedule was frenetic—often touring several bases a day. Most celebrities travelled north, and huge audiences watched Bob Hope and other "headliners." We were grateful for the few who ventured to the delta. Efrem was friendly but offered no personal views of the war. He confirmed my suspicion they were briefed of "appropriate" topics to discuss with soldiers. I understood but wanted to know the sentiments of entertainers and views of the public. The war was becoming more controversial. We relied on press releases and letters from home, but our data were limited. After lunch Zimbalist left to see two additional units before nightfall.

The day was calm, as both Gen. Minh and Col. Maddow were absent. Although it rained, the temperature remained high. Vinh and Woodruff performed three surgeries and discussed their trip to Saigon as they enjoyed a 33 beer. Vinh had taken Bill to a Chinese opera. During the performance a bomb exploded in the foyer. They remembered the bomb more than the opera. On their return flight the 'bou's landing gear failed to function and the pilot circled the field as he struggled with the controls. Eventually, they landed without incident, but it was a fitting climax of an exciting trip for the two Bac Si's.

Sp5 Chambers joined our MILPHAP team. He had been in VN for six months and seen considerable action in the north. Another new member was Co Trien, an interpreter. She lived in Bac Lieu for several years but had been working with a special forces medical research team at Can Tho. Of Chinese extraction, she spoke several Chinese dialects as well as Cambodian, French, and Vietnamese. Our interpreters now included Co Phung, Co Tuyet, Mr. Thai, Mr. Ky, Co Trien, and Co Ha, secretary. One referred to young single women as Co, whereas married or older females were addressed as Ba.

The "Committee of Responsibility" (COR) visited Bac Lieu. The COR was a private group of U.S. citizens concerned with children's casualties. The touring members included an administrator and three physicians. We provided hospital statistics as they photographed hospital staff and patients. Dr. Vinh was interviewed and patiently answered their questions. The group was pleasantly surprised by the quality of care and were encouraged to learn we treated all war victims, especially children. They visited many hospitals throughout the country.

COR was formed in New York by physicians and activists alarmed by the plight of VN civilians, particularly children. To understand the magnitude of the problem, a group toured 35 provincial hospitals in 1967, the team that met with us. They reported up to 60 percent of war injuries involved children, like other estimates. Following their visit to VN, COR determined the best method to provide care was to evacuate children to America, a daunting task. The goal was hampered by both VN and American bureaucracy, and only 100 children were ultimately transported to the states; nearly all returned to VN. COR was supported and sponsored by prominent peace activists, including Dr. Benjamin Spock, Julie Andrews, Coretta Scott King, and Mrs. Eugene McCarthy. Although COR was dissolved in 1974, it maintained a field office in Saigon until 1978.

Dr. Vinh called to his office to thank me for help obtaining his new TV set and items I purchased for him in Japan. As he spoke, a worker placed a large wicker basket in his office which held a neatly coiled nine-foot reticulated python. Vinh said the snake was "domesticated," although I approached it with caution, as I'd seen bites by "nonvenomous" snakes. The snake was indeed tame, as it did not object to being handled, happily coiling over the shoulders of anyone brave enough to pick up the 40-pound serpent. But when a chicken was placed in its cage for weekly feeding, the snake quickly swallowed the hapless bird, which became a bulge in the snake's body. Vinh had workers erect a cage adjacent to my hooch, and the snake became an attraction as MACV officers eagerly posed for pictures with the reptile.

Evening call had become routine—two or three injured by a mine, mortar, or aircraft, plus a patient or two with intestinal infections or pneumonia, an attempted suicide, and usually a maternity call. As I walked to the hospital a full moon was visible and the night was balmy. The moonlight brightened several rows of stratocumulus clouds and cast sufficient light to read. The beauty of the scene was marred by the nightly artillery salvos.

After the moon came the rain—the trail to the hospital was a continuous four-inch puddle of mud and slime—no sandals on call!

We were warned of a VC attack, as May Day would be celebrated throughout the communist world. A lightning bug patrolled overhead, and Tom Needham was aboard a chopper that received several machine gun rounds. Defenses were fortified throughout the compound.

The following evening, I was summoned to the maternity ward by an urgent note: "Please see 21-year girl with bleeding—Fell from bridge last night—No pregnant—no married." When I examined the distraught girl, I found a large vaginal laceration. The midwives were amused and tittering to one another, but the girl was in tears. She had been sexually assaulted. The midwives made no attempt to locate the offender or call the police. I repaired the defect and left, confused and depressed; why had the midwives not reported the rape?

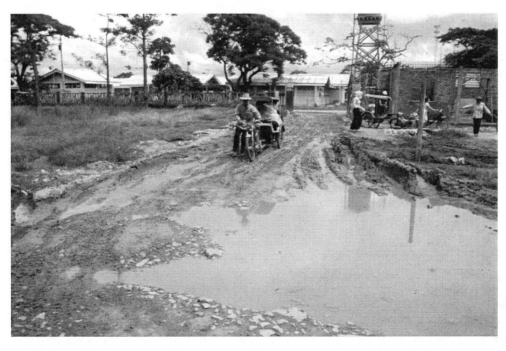

Muddy hospital road.

Jim Jones had been ill for the past few days and was jaundiced. Steve arranged a dust off to the 93rd Evac Hospital for workup. We feared he had hepatitis.

Medical knowledge of hepatitis was expanding rapidly in the mid–1960s. Two forms of hepatitis had been identified: infectious hepatitis, or "epidemic jaundice," now known as hepatitis A, transmitted by contaminated food and water; and Hepatitis B, or serum hepatitis, spread by blood, or injections, including IV drug abuse, or sexual contact. Most cases among American troops were infectious hepatitis. Beginning 1966, incoming combat soldiers were given gamma globulin (GG) prophylaxis. This didn't extend to MILPHAP physicians as neither Jim, Charlie, nor I received GG, and the practice was limited to troops with high risk. The disease was common and thousands of American troops were infected. Prolonged bed rest was advocated to prevent potentially fatal complications with significant loss of duty. However, a large study at Cam Ranh Bay revealed moderate activity was safe and led to more rapid convalescence and earlier return to duty. Hepatitis B was less common, usually related to parenteral drug abuse, and became to a greater problem as the war progressed.

Following the war many VN veterans developed Hepatitis C, a form of hepatitis unknown during the 1960s, but an important cause of liver failure, cancer, and other complications. The 2020 Nobel prize was awarded to three researchers who discovered Hepatitis C.

We believed Jim had hepatitis A, or infectious hepatitis. The duration of his confinement was unknown. If he were evacuated to the States our physician group would be diminished by one-third. I called Dr. Marsh for a replacement if Jim's absence were prolonged.

An operation near Ca Mau killed 75 VC. A pilot was wounded, and Steve treated the officer. A machine gun bullet smashed the Huey's plexiglass canopy and traversed up the pilot's leg as it damaged his shin. The slug ended its trajectory in his flak jacket, without any chest injury.

We received no news of Jim's condition but a call from Can Tho reassured me if Jim required evacuation, we would receive a replacement. Meanwhile, a new AMA volunteer physician would join us within a few days, a general practitioner.

A C-123, known as a "pregnant caribou" or "thunder-pig," landed at Bac Lieu with the medical equipment from Columbo. The C-123 was the largest aircraft our strip could accommodate. The plane looked like a larger version of the Canadian 'bou, but was built by Fairchild aviation, an American company. The two-engine craft carried a large payload of 25,000 pounds and could take off and land on a 1,000' runway. In addition to carrying cargo, planes were modified for defoliation as well as flare ships. A related but larger aircraft, the C-130 Lockheed Hercules, was a four-engine turboprop with a payload of more than 40,000 pounds.

These aircraft have been confused with the Douglas C-47, the two-engine military version of the DC-3, which dated from World War II. The C-47 was modified with multiple weapons to become "Spooky" or "Puff the Magic Dragon."

An Air America Beechcraft brought our new AMA volunteer physician, Dr. William Harris. A handsome, outgoing chap in his mid–30s, Bill graduated from the UC School of Medicine and worked as a generalist at the same Kaiser facility as

Dr. Woodruff, who told his California colleague of his duties and challenges during lunch. Harris was a confirmed vegetarian and vegan, although he had no difficulties selecting his menu as he disarmed officers with his easy going affect. Bill was eager to begin work in the hospital.

I assisted Dr. Vinh on a difficult surgery for gastric carcinoma. As we waited for the next patient to be prepped, Vinh was in a reflective mood. He asked of my trip to Japan and spoke knowingly of the country as he recounted a popular parable in the Orient: "There are four criteria for a successful life: marry a Japanese woman; eat Chinese food; drive an American car, and sleep in a French bed." He had accomplished none of these criteria except eating Chinese food but was happy and felt he lived a good life. Vinh smiled knowingly as the nurse indicated the next case was ready. We scrubbed and donned new surgical gowns.

Jim called from the Evac Hospital, confirming he had infectious hepatitis. He would be hospitalized for another week, followed by transfer to Vung Tau for convalescence, with return to Bac Lieu a few weeks later.

That evening Maj. Aguilar took the MILPHAP doctors to the 105 mm howitzer gun emplacement to view the nightly H&I fire. Finally, we would observe the source of the noise we endured each night. We were ushered through a gate to the two weapons, a stone's throw from the MACV compound, and to the fire direction control (FDC) bunker. Inside the FDC a large map was spread over a wooden table. Friendly forces were marked with blue grease pencil, identifying patrols, ranger units, and ARVN platoons. Small red "X's" designated suspected VC positions. The evening's targets were numbered, and their coordinates plotted. The gun crew chief said the range of the guns was approximately 10,000 meters, depending on the charge. The 75 mm recoilless rifles had a maximum range of 7,000 meters, giving the ARVN considerable advantage. The 105s in Bac Lieu and nearby ARVN outposts also had overlapping coverage, although there were gaps which the VC exploited. Atop the covered villa that served as the site's headquarters, a soldier watched for flashes of VC mortars

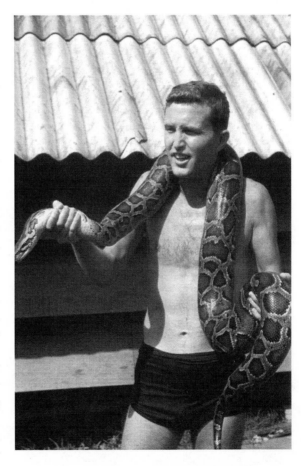

Dr. Bill Harris and author's python.

or recoilless rifles. Additional spotters were located throughout Bac Lieu and communicated with the FDC by radio. American bases had sophisticated radar arrays integrated with the howitzers and could pinpoint a target and automatically return fire within two minutes. Such hi-tech equipment was not available to ARVN gunners, who relied on visual sightings and plotting targets by hand.

The chief's comments were interrupted as the guns commenced firing. We walked outside as the weapons broke the darkness with each blast. From the end of the barrel, four or five feet of flame belched forth each time the howitzer roared. The crew were firing charge 6 loads—the next to maximum charge. Each shell was nearly three feet long and weighed more than 40 pounds. The projectile was more than a foot in length and contained several pounds of high explosives. Projectiles were adaptable for armor or cement penetration, antipersonnel or chemical (such as phosphorus).

The chief explained the various fuses that controlled the time when the explosive charge would detonate. I recalled the recent fatal accident due to a misfire of a variable time (VT) fuse, killing one of their comrades. Although we held our ears as they fired, the guns were not as loud as we experienced from the MACV compound. But we were standing behind the guns, which shot over the compound, increasing the noise.

105 mm howitzer.

The 105 mm howitzer is a mobile cannon that has been a staple of several armies for decades. Modern howitzers originated in Europe more than 200 years ago and were typically short-barreled cannons. The weapons were employed extensively in World Wars I and II. The guns used in VN were often mounted on a moveable carriage and could be trailed by a jeep. Larger caliber guns, 155 mm, could also be transported by vehicle.

Chapter Sources

Gunter Levy. *America in Vietnam*. Oxford: Oxford University Press, 1978.

E. M. Kennedy. "Civilian War Casualties in Vietnam." Congressional Record: Senate. December 22, 1969. Washington, D.C.: U.S. Government Printing Office, S17508.

H. A. F. Dudley, R. J. Knight, J. C. McNeur, et al. "Civilian Battle Casualties in South Vietnam." *British Journal of Surgery* 55, no. 5 (1968): 332–40.

United States Senate Committee on the Judiciary, Subcommittee on Problems Connected with Refugees and Escapees, War-Related Civilian Problems in Indochina. Part 1. Vietnam, Hearing, 92nd Congress 1st Session 21, Print 50–8110, p. 475. Washington, D.C.: U.S. Government Printing Office, April 1971.

United States Senate Committee on the Judiciary, Subcommittee to Investigate Problems Connected with

Refugees and Escapees: Refugees and Civilian War Casualty Problems in Indochina: A Staff Report. Committee Print 50-S110. Washington, D.C.: U.S. Government Printing Office, 1970.

E. A. Vaslyan. "Civilian War Casualties and Medical Care in South Vietnam." *Annals of Internal Medicine* 74, no. 4 (1971): 611–24.

Spurgeon Neel. "Preventive Medicine" and "Summary." Chapters 8 and 14 in *Medical Support of the U.S. Army in Vietnam 1965–1970.* Washington, D.C.: U.S. Government Printing Office, 1973.

Myron Allukian, Jr., and Paul L. Atwood. "The Vietnam War." In *War and Public Health.* Edited by Barry S. Levy and Victor W. Sidel. Oxford Scholarship Online, 2009.

"Committee of Responsibility." *New York Times.* February 2, 1967.

Committee of Responsibility. Swarthmore College Peace Collection DG-73.

Joe A. Dean and Andre J. Ognibene. "Hepatitis." Chapter 18 in *Internal Medicine in Vietnam, Vol. II: General Medicine and Infectious Diseases.* Edited by Andre J. Ognibene and O'Neill Barrett, Jr., Washington, D.C.: U.S. Government Printing Office, 1982.

Stanley Karnow. "Giap Remembers." *New York Times Magazine,* June 24, 1990.

Jay H. Hoofnagle and Stephen M. Feinstone. "The Discovery of Hepatitis C: The 2020 Nobel Prize in Physiology and Medicine." *New England Journal of Medicine* 383, no. 24 (2020): 2297–99.

Raymond S. Koff and Kurt J. Isselbacher. "Changing Concepts in the Epidemiology of Viral Hepatitis." *New England Journal of Medicine* 278, no. 25 (1968): 1371–80.

Saul Krugman, Robert Ward, and Joan P. Giles. "Natural History of Infectious Hepatitis." *American Journal of Medicine* 32, no. 5 (1962): 717–28.

Robert W. McCollum. "The Elusive Etiologic Agents of Viral Hepatitis." *American Journal of Public Health Nations Health* 53, no. 10 (1963): 1630–4.

Susan F. Sullivan and A. J. Zuckerman. "Viral Hepatitis in Drug Addicts." *Postgraduate Medical Journal* 47, no. 549 (1971): 473–5.

10

May

Fear, a Round in the Whore House

I began the second half of my allotted time in Vietnam. The anniversary didn't occur to me as I methodically pursued my now familiar hospital duties, oblivious to activities elsewhere in the country. The marines were fighting another bloody battle at Khe Sanh in I Corps, but warfare in the DTA was surreal. MACV officers rose, ate breakfast in the mess hall, then rode choppers to battle where they advised their Vietnamese colleagues. The men returned to the compound's comfort for dinner or BBQ, drinks, and a movie. Occasionally, fighting would persist for two days, requiring Americans to bivouac in the field overnight with their Vietnamese colleagues. The loss of an advisor or pilot was an infrequent but somber event in the delta, but injury and death were omnipresent for those fighting elsewhere in the country.

In the evenings, Steve and MACV officers recounted thrilling, often poignant stories of battle. I recorded the events, experiencing the war vicariously; but the results were real, a never-ending cascade of injured and dead, matched by VC violence. The advisors were dedicated soldiers, but their life differed markedly from American fighting men in northern combat units.

News from the States was difficult to interpret from our delta perspective. Opposition to the war mounted, although the U.S. government remained steadfast. In early May, General Westmoreland was warmly received by a joint session of Congress as he requested more money and troops. B-52 bombers had completed 10,000 bombing missions, raining 200,000 tons of ordnance on the enemy. Life in Bac Lieu had become a familiar pattern, although this was soon to be shattered by more danger and fear.

May 1, Workers Day of the World, was a holiday and the hospital was closed except for emergency procedures. Following the morning surgery schedule, the MILPHAP physicians met in Vinh's office. He was in an expansive mood and regaled us with tales of Dalat.

For more than a century French and wealthy Vietnamese have fled Saigon's heat and humidity to the mountain retreat. Dalat has been compared to the Alps, with pine forests, lakes, and a mild climate. Pheasants and peacocks are native, as well as a variety of big game animals.

Dalat was discovered by Dr. Alexandre Yersin (1863–1943), the Albert Schweitzer of Vietnam. Yersin became famous for his work with plague, and the organism now bears his name: *Yerseni pestis*, previously termed for his mentor, Pasteur, *Pasteurella pestis*.

After medical training and research with Pasteur, Yersin travelled to Hong Kong where he discovered the plague bacteria. He subsequently made his way to Indochina, tramping through jungles on a walking tour from Nha Trang to Dalat, site of the Vietnamese Pasteur Institute, which he founded. He also initiated the medical school in Hanoi. All Vietnamese revere Yersin, who died during World War II and is buried near Dalat. There are no monuments to the good doctor, but Dr. Vinh assured us his memory is safely preserved.

Vinh reminisced about some of his Dalat hunting adventures. He exclaimed, "It is gibler [bountiful]. One can shoot squirrels, monkeys, tiger, elephant, peacocks, deer, and many birds, plus gaur [a type of buffalo]. In the streams and lakes are many fish. The VN say, 'Co nuoc thi, so co ca'—where there is water there are fish. And the forest has many animals." He said hunting in Dalat was exciting, but could be hazardous, not just for tigers, but even monkeys. He once shot the leader of a monkey tribe. The other monkeys were angry and chased him, throwing stones. He gestured excitedly, "Very dangerous—I ran and shot over my shoulder as I fled." With that finale, Vinh promised to take us to Dalat. We nodded politely and retreated to the compound for a nap.

Dr. Vinh hosted a farewell dinner for Dr. Woodruff, another multicourse French meal with wine and cognac, followed by Mrs. Vinh's vocal selections. Bill applauded warmly and gave Mrs. Vinh a hug. The party concluded early because of a curfew.

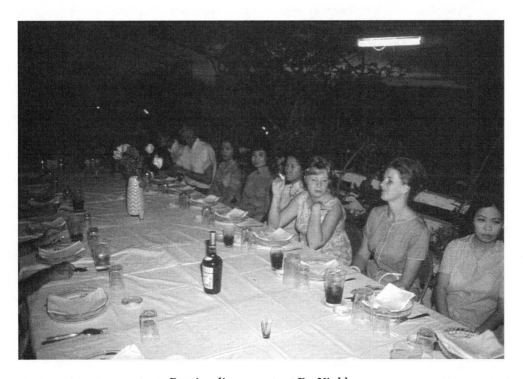

Evening dinner party at Dr. Vinh's.

Despite a busy surgical schedule, Dr. Vinh escorted Bill Woodruff to the airport where the surgeon boarded the morning 'bou. Woodruff was an excellent surgeon, friend, a great asset who made a lasting impression on Vinh.

William Woodruff graduated from Duke University School of Medicine in 1940 and entered the military. He also served in Korea, followed by a successful practice with the California Kaiser group (William Woodruff, MD, 1914–2000).

VC violence near Gia Rai injured four children aged 2–10 years, with fragment wounds of the face and extremities—two lost eyes. Another two boys sustained fractures. Despite their plight, the children seemed to accept their fate, although it was heartbreaking to round on these kids. To see their eye wounds was devastating. As we completed surgery, four patients arrived from Lung Lom, claiming their water supply had been poisoned by a substance dropped from an airplane. All had symptoms of severe gastroenteritis and dehydration. One girl died on arrival. The others recovered with aggressive fluid therapy. Vinh sent a relative to obtain water samples for testing. I checked with tactical operations center (TOC) and learned no choppers or airplanes had recently flown defoliation or chemical operations. The TOC memo included the false statement from Saigon briefings that defoliants were harmless, and chemical operations were always preceded by psy-war planes and leaflets. However, the TOC correctly indicated chemicals were used sparingly in the delta, primarily in the U Minh forest.

I asked Vinh if we could visit the area, but he said it was controlled by VC and unsafe. A few days later we received the water samples. Dr. Vinh sent a portion to the Pasteur Institute and I forwarded another to USAID for analysis.

I held MACV sick call for Steve who was ill with fever, chills, and body aches. His temperature was 104 degrees, and we loaded him onto a dust off to the 36th Evac Hospital. I thought he might have scrub typhus, or dengue fever. Our medical group was rapidly becoming decimated by disease.

Scrub typhus is due to a unique Rickettsia microorganism by the bite of a mite or chigger found in grassy or brushy terrain. The disease was identified in the 3rd century BCE in China. Scrub typhus has a colorful name, Tsutsugamushi fever, from the Japanese word "dangerous mite." The disease is endemic in Vietnam and troops deployed in densely foliated regions were frequently infected. Although scrub typhus did not lead to any U.S. deaths, it accounted for 20–30 percent of FUOs, or fever of unknown origin, among soldiers and was probably underreported. Scrub typhus was uncommon in the delta, but Steve may have contracted it during an ARVN operation in the U Minh forest.

More rain—if the VC shelled us, we'd have to wade to the bunkers. Despite the mud, clinics were busy. At 1:00 p.m. we saw B-52 bombers flying to Cambodia for "carpet-bombing." In clinic a lady presented with advanced leprosy. Her fingers and toes were nearly destroyed, together with the classic "leonine" faces. Several leprosy patients resided in the "old people" building behind the hospital.

Leprosy dates to antiquity, and in biblical times "lepers" were shunned because of their skin lesions and disfigurement, although many lepers described in the bible likely suffered from other diseases: psoriasis, fungal infections, or other dermal lesions. The disease causes painless ulcers, especially on the face, which evolve to the "leonine" lesions. The organism also attacks the peripheral nervous system, with loss of digits and deformities.

Leprosy is a chronic infection due to a bacterium related to tuberculosis, *Mycobacterium leprae*, identified by the Norwegian physician Gerhard Hansen in 1868. The disease is often called "Hansen's disease." Leprosy is not very contagious, usually requiring prolonged contact, although the disease is relatively common in Vietnam. Despite lack of contact with U.S. troops, several cases were identified among American soldiers, with sporadic reports in veterans. We observed many skin lesions we could not diagnose that our VN colleagues believed were leprosy. A recent VN government program has led to a dramatic decline in prevalence.

There was a huge rainstorm and water was above the floor in several hooches.

Rain did not deter the enemy. VC attacked a reconnaissance company within 4 km of Bac Lieu, killing four ARVN soldiers, provoking a brisk artillery response. Another attack was feared, and we lay awake, poised to run to our bunker with flashlight, medical kit, and helmet, another sleepless night with heavy H&I cannonade. Sleep had become an issue and "siesta" time each afternoon was now reserved for a nap.

Brushing aside fatigue at 1:00 a.m., I walked through the mud to the hospital to examine a 21-year-old woman who had surgery for an ectopic pregnancy two days

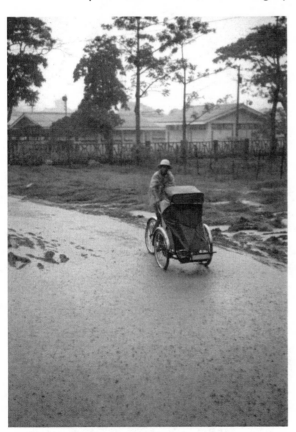

earlier. She was short of breath and coughing bloody secretions with a rapid, thready pulse. I thought she suffered from either a pulmonary embolism (clot) or a lung infection and gave her antibiotics and a transfusion. We had no methods to diagnose or treat a pulmonary embolism. Despite our rudimentary diagnostic and therapeutic tools, she improved by afternoon.

Col. Maddox introduced me to the inspector general (IG) who was auditing the compound. The IG asked me about my team and the hospital, but Col. Maddox interrupted, providing all the responses. The IG wasn't satisfied and requested a tour. His son was an MSC officer, and the IG was keenly interested in medical issues. I was pleased as he said our facility was better than most province hospitals he had seen.

Children playing outside

Delivering a patient in the rain.

the ER invented a new toy. They found a large beetle and fashioned a wire framework around a small metal car. Pinning the wings back, they connected the insect to the car with a paperclip. As the beetle beat its wings, it moved the car forward, an ingenious device. All one needed was a ready supply of insects, of which we had no shortage!

Mariana returned on the 'bou from her Japan R&R with Dr. Alan Homay, our newest AMA physician to offset our doctor shortage. Homay was a sprightly, greying man of 47 years, born and educated in Iran, who lived in Switzerland before coming to the United States. He was a general practitioner with a wide experience. Importantly, he spoke fluent French, to Vinh's delight, who met him in the afternoon.

Dr. Khoung referred a girl with suspected diphtheria to clinic. She had a throat infection but did not appear very toxic. I'd never seen diphtheria, so we isolated her and sent a throat culture to Can Tho.

The report on the suspected poisoned water revealed no poisons or toxins but had marked bacterial growth. Perhaps the citizens were not poisoned, but victims of poor sanitation. I remained suspicious of their malady but never learned the cause.

Steve returned from Vung Tau, recovered from his illness. His final diagnosis was FUO, but doctors suspected he had dengue fever. After four days of fluids and observation, his condition improved, and he was discharged. He felt weak but otherwise well.

Dengue fever is an arbor-virus (arthropod-borne) transmitted by the *Aedes aegypti* mosquito. The disease has affected military operations for hundreds of years in Asia, especially during World War II. Dengue is also known as "breakbone fever" and hemorrhagic complications may be fatal. Dengue accounted for many FUOs in VN and was second only to venereal disease for days lost from military duty. As Steve's illness, the average confinement was four to five days. A vaccine is now available.

Dr. Homay began hospital duties, promptly arriving

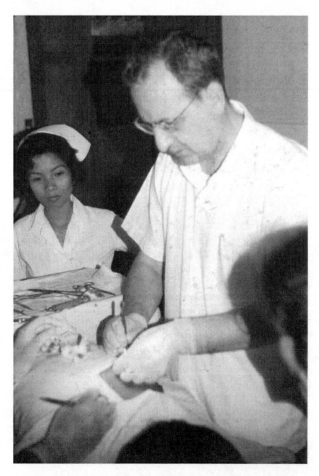

VN nurse and Dr. Homay operating on trauma victim—possible VC.

at 7:15 a.m. The clinic was not open, and he waited on the steps, playing with the ever-present children. He made maternity and surgical rounds and visited the orphanage with Mariana.

The orphanage remained a depressing place. The nuns asked for scraps of wood to build coffins. "Fine or expensive wood is not necessary," they told her. "Anything will do." They had been forced to use cardboard boxes for the tiny corpses, not ideal during the rainy season.

A bizarre, ghastly accident occurred on a canal near Gia Rai. A young woman was attempting to start one of the long-shaft outboard motors on her sampan. She pulled repeatedly at the starter rope, but the engine refused to turn over. Undaunted, she stood at the stern of the small wooden boat and gave one last tug. The engine started but she lost her balance and fell backwards. Her hair became ensnarled in the engine's starter rope assembly, and within seconds she was completely scalped. She was found by a passing boat and taken to Gia Rai. Her scalp was retrieved. A U.S. medic clamped bleeding vessels and transported her to Bac Lieu. In the ER she was completely lucid despite massive loss of blood. We gave fluids, controlled the bleeding sites, and cleaned her skull as we tried to reattach the scalp. Neither Charlie nor I could recall survival after scalping in tales of the wild west and feared blood supply to the reattached scalp would be inadequate.

Amazingly, the woman remained awake and without complaints despite obvious pain; her family was unaware of the grave situation.

The scalping was accompanied by two deaths on maternity. Charlie admitted a woman with a severe uterine infection (amnionitis) who died within an hour. He

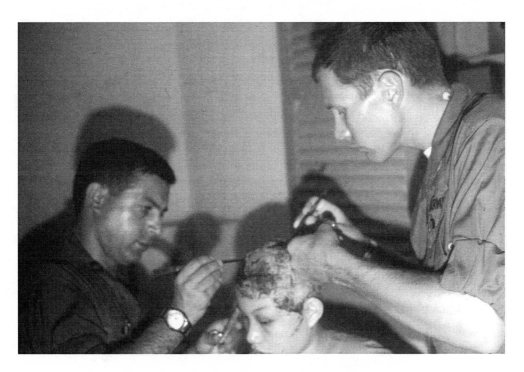

Dr. Charlie Gueriera, scalped victim, and author.

performed an emergency postmortem C-section to rescue the baby but was unsuccessful. Another pregnant woman died of typhoid fever. The husband was grief stricken, with no funds for a coffin or to transport her body home. One of the ward staff gave him 200 piastres for a cyclo, and the lifeless form was loaded onto the contraption.

We held a big loop clinic, as Pat, Ba Thao, and I placed 20 IUDs. Two women returned to clinic, requesting their devices be removed as their husbands decided to have more children. More than 150 IUDs had been placed since the program's onset, and news was rapidly spreading of the service. Perhaps there was too much publicity, as we soon learned.

Not all Bac Lieu events were serious—some were comical, although not for all participants. Mr. Hayes, the USAID officer, held a cocktail party and dinner. The chief of police and several prominent citizens were present as well as Charlie, Vinh, and I. When we arrived, the party was in full swing, including one man who quickly recognized Charlie. The thin, bespectacled chap in his mid–50s with an open print shirt and drink in hand rushed to him, embracing Charlie as he spoke rapidly in Vietnamese. It seems Charlie had cured his grandson of some malady and the man wanted to show his appreciation to the Italian-American Bac Si. He insisted Charlie sit across from him and swapped toasts as we awaited dinner, which proved to be a marathon drinking bout by the Vietnamese gentleman. Midway through dinner the man passed out and was carried to his car by his friends as we watched with amusement. Cognac, wine, and whiskey don't mix!

Dr. Marsh called to inform me a Stanford medical student will join us for three months. I was impressed a medical student would volunteer for Vietnam.

In the morning we examined the scalped patient, who was stable, but it was too early to know if grafts would be successful. After instructions for her care, Charlie and I caught the 'bou to Vung Tau to visit Jim.

As our plane glided over the water on final approach, I saw hundreds of ships and boats waiting to be unloaded. Two jetties and deep-water berths had been built since my last visit and the port was bustling. Helicopters of all types, as well as Mohawks, Caribous, Skyraiders, C123s, C130s, and other aircraft lined the strips, and there were acres of cars, trucks, and other vehicles parked on adjacent dunes. New construction was everywhere, including billets, warehouses, and offices. Vung Tau had become a major logistical site for the war.

We walked to the 36th Evac Hospital, a series of Quonset huts, and found Jim in an air-conditioned ward with other hepatitis patients. He said he would be released in a week, although he wasn't authorized to go to the beach.

One of the first army hospitals to be opened in VN was the 8th Field Hospital in Saigon, a 100-bed facility, supplemented by a Saigon Naval dispensary in 1963. In 1965, the army began a major expansion of medical facilities, adopting the concept of initial medical and surgical management, with evacuation if treatment required more than 30 days of hospitalization. By December 1965, bed capacity in Vietnam exceeded 1,600, with construction the following year of four surgical hospitals, six evacuation hospitals and another field hospital. These buildouts included the 36th Evac Hospital in Vung Tau, which began service in 1966. Total bed capacity exceeded

5,000 by the 1970s. From 1965 and 1970, 133,000 wounded were treated, with nearly 100,00 hospital admissions. Mortality was 2.6 percent, one-half that of World War II. Improved survival was credited to rapid helicopter evacuation and extensive use of blood products and IV fluids, together with advanced surgical expertise and medical support.

Survival from war's trauma in VN was substantially improved compared to that of World War II or Korea, despite high velocity injuries and multiple sites of injury. Incremental gains were achieved in Iraq and Afghanistan. But the total number of U.S. casualties in VN was approximately 47,000, compared to 4,000 for Iraq and 1,800 for Afghanistan. Unfortunately, improvements in surgical technique and medical management have been exceeded by an even greater severity of wounds for the Middle East conflicts.

Significant medical research was conducted in Vietnam. Teams from Walter Reed and other facilities studied "shock lung," or post-traumatic pulmonary insufficiency, and cholera, plague, malaria, dengue fever, melioidosis, and other illnesses, including psychological aspects of combat stress—later to be termed post-traumatic stress disorder, or PTSD.

Charlie and I checked into the Huong Hotel. After a French dinner at Cyrano's restaurant, we strolled downtown. I was struck by the blatant, wide-open atmosphere. Bars were everywhere. Curbside girls literally dragged soldiers inside. We saw bars, girls, drunks, fights, curio shops, and more bars. The scene was more raucous and bawdier than Saigon. The town was filled with EMs on R&R as well as soldiers stationed in Vung Tau who could secure a live-in girl, which often led to trouble. One recent tragic incident involved a sergeant with a wife and children in the States, plus a VN girlfriend. A week before the soldier was to rotate home, the girl's boyfriend arrived and found her with the soldier. The man dragged her into the street and a fight ensued. The American knocked the boyfriend down, upon which he pulled a .45 pistol and shot the sergeant in the head, killing him instantly.

Most of the girls who worked in Vung Tau's bars were 15–17 years old, managed by bar owners, usually women (mamasons), who provided the girls a place to live and paid them for work in the bar, plus other "duties." Many of the young girls were pretty, but a few had already attained the professional "hooker" appearance. At the Grand Hotel, girls were expensive: 120 piastres for a 15-minute glass of Saigon tea. To take a girl "all night" was 2,000–3,000 piastres (20 to 30 U.S. dollars). In the smaller clubs the girls cost less. Hotels did not allow a girl into a GI's room without an ID card, which was left at the front desk, along with a tip for the hotel. At the end of the interlude the ID card was returned. If anything was stolen or lost, the hotel could trace the girl. There were numerous streetwalkers as well, but the main business was conducted by "bar girls." The term "streetwalker" isn't accurate, as most were "motorcycle-riders," drumming up business as they rode on Hondas and Suzukis driven by their pimp boyfriends.

Three beautiful sandy beaches adorned Vung Tau, although undertows and riptides could be dangerous, with 27 drownings in three months. The beaches were crowded with GIs and featured concession stands for food and beer. Vietnamese children also walked the sand, hawking fresh pineapple, fruits, and souvenirs.

It was windy but the water pleasantly warm. We saw one man tended by life-guards for a jelly fish sting. Some envenomations could be life threatening.

The next morning, we took the bus to the airport. Our 'bou took off promptly, but one engine sputtered and was feathered, and we returned to Vung Tau for repairs. Within an hour we were again in the air but the engine again failed. The third time was not the charm—the engine malfunctioned and the plane was grounded. Charlie and I spent another night in Vung Tau.

The following morning it was raining when we boarded the airport bus. As we sat on a bench, the rain stopped and the runway and dunes steamed in the morning sun. Nearby an old Ba with two gold front teeth picked up cigarette butts and trash that littered the area, placing them in a dixie cup. She dutifully collected the rubbish, her blouse soaked by the rain, displaying a cheap, soggy foam bra. Soldiers discarded additional candy wrappers and cigarette butts as they waited. This didn't offend the Ba: as long as Americans left trash, she would have a job.

The Caribou loaded and we reclined among tractor tires, fan belts, and cases of condensed milk. There were no malfunctions, and we arrived a few hours later in Bac Lieu, another tale of the Army's "hurry up to wait."

The 105s awoke us at 4:00 a.m. with an early morning fusillade in response to a VC attack of an outpost three miles from town by mortars, recoilless rifles, and small arms. Four ARVN were wounded, and the structure demolished. We received several civilian casualties and another two from Vinh Chau. The war continued.

It was the eve of Ho Chi Minh's birthday and Vinh was fearful of an attack. He did not operate, warning, "Tonight is bad—I stay in my home."

We prayed the rumors were false. Gia Rai officials were concerned, as propaganda leaflets threatened violence.

The night lasted forever. Ho Chi Minh's birthday was heralded by continuous ARVN artillery shelling as lightship choppers buzzed overhead, with Spookys waiting. The lightning bugs cast their several million candle-power-beams earthbound like a silver line in the sky, an upside-down searchlight. Air strikes rocked our hooch. Many officers wore shoes or boots to bed, with helmets at their side. But the VC did not attack.

Bill Harris and Charlie treated a mother and two-year-old son shot near Soc Trang by a chopper. They had reached the main highway and flagged a passing bus. The mother had a neck wound and her child was shot in the face.

A divisional operation near Vi Thang was a military failure but produced many casualties. No VC contact was made, but ARVN soldiers tripped booby traps, killing several.

Johnny Grant, a Los Angeles radio personality, visited the compound, interviewing LA residents, including Steve and me for later broadcast.

A curfew was in place and Bac Lieu was off-limits.

Although the VC didn't shell Bac Lieu for Ho Chi Minh's birthday, they caused mischief elsewhere. In Vinh Chau they hit an outpost, kidnapped and assassinated two hamlet officials, then detonated several mines. We admitted four victims, including two young men shot by the lightning bug. I did not question their allegiance. They remained on the ward for two days then disappeared.

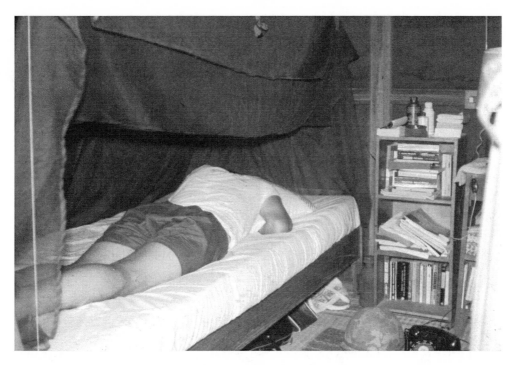

Sleeping with helmet ready in hooch.

The second day's operation was more successful: 95 VC killed with two ARVN fatalities. Measuring military success by body count was now routine, a macabre technique.

The chief of police asked Charlie and me to join him at the ARVN officers' club for dancing and drinking. We listened to a six-member band play stilted American numbers as officers, wives, and friends moved about the floor under a moon-lit night. Charlie danced with the wife of Gen. Minh's chief-of-staff, Col. Diem. As the band played, a large gecko crawled across the whitewashed wall behind the drummer, uttering its odd-sounding cries. Bats flew in and out of the rafters, carrying insects to their babies. It was a scene from a 1940s movie—I expected Alan Ladd to emerge in trench coat from the shadows. Artillery fired a few rounds, but the blasts were subdued for the party. Flags and decorations had been put up around town to celebrate Buddha's birthday, or Christmas of the Orient, as Vinh called it. Our festivities

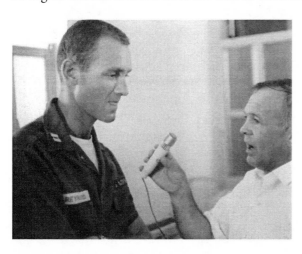

Dr. Steve Reynard interviewed by Los Angeles radio announcer Johnny Grant.

were interrupted at 10:00 p.m., when a messenger handed me a note—a typhoid abdominal perforation and an ectopic pregnancy awaited Vinh and me.

Smiling prisoners performed various chores around the compound under the watchful eyes of their ARVN guards, repairing bunkers' rotten timbers and adding new sandbags. As they toiled, guards forced them to sing the VN national anthem, a humiliating task. But, no sing, no work! As their lyrical efforts drifted over the compound, it was clear their hearts were not into choir duty.

Although we didn't hear or see it, a lightning bug was above Bac Lieu last evening. The aircraft received automatic weapons fire from several sources, which was returned by gunships. At breakfast Jean Reed told me the night's melee was violent and warned we would receive casualties. He was correct. Later that morning a teenage girl was brought from a VC-controlled area. She had been shot by a helicopter as she assisted VC fighters. Her wounds were severe, and she was in dire straits, short of breath and cyanotic. One lung had been hit. A VC doctor had attended her other wounds but did not address the chest injury. Charlie and I put in a chest tube, which improved her breathing. I was surprised when she smiled as we finished the procedure.

It was warm, 105 degrees in the hooch with both fans running, and too hot to sunbathe. Several of us took turns turning the crank on an ice cream machine. After an hour of work, we sampled our homemade vanilla ice cream—delicious! An hour later we wore ponchos as we barbecued steaks at the Paddy Rat Lounge barbecue. The sun shone through the clouds, but the rain wasn't impeded. The scene reminded me of a California beach party.

Bill Harris treated a never-ending stream of ER patients during his call. The girl with the chest tube improved but we'd been unable to obtain a transfusion. The scalp victim was spiking a high fever and delirious.

Jim wrote the University of California San Francisco (UCSF), requesting a surgical refresher program for Dr. Vinh. I made a similar request of USC.

Several airstrikes lit the evening sky that was also illuminated by lightning bugs and there was small arms fire nearby. An officer in the next hooch was playing Tchaikovsky's 1812 Overture, the cannons in the piece blending with the howitzers.

The music was a prelude to a terrifying evening, as the VC focused their weapons on the compound. After typing my journal entry, I put away the typewriter, grabbed toothbrush, and walked to the latrine. I stepped out of the building at 11:45 p.m. There was no sound except the diesel generator. A nearly full moon had a ring around it and the hooches were dark. As I turned the corner, I heard the unmistakable sound of a 75 mm—a short, high-pitched whizz immediately followed by a loud crack. Incoming rounds! Within seconds I was in our bunker, followed by Don as a second round exploded nearby. Soon the bunker was full of crouched forms, panting and cursing a stubbed toe, forgotten cigarettes, or a fall into the ditch. Luckily, no one was seriously injured. The rounds continued, some very close, raining debris on the bunker's roof. I was grateful for the recent repair. The explosions were soon answered by ARVN artillery. More than 200 rounds peppered VC positions.

The 75s continued firing at us, punctuating the sky with flashes of light as we huddled on the bunker's sandy floor. By the blasts' glow I looked across at new officers, fear written on their faces. I was scared, but less terrified, as the awful events were now familiar to me.

At the dawn of the 20th century the eminent Harvard physiologist Walter Cannon began his classic studies of stress and danger, publishing books and scientific papers over a span of several decades. Cannon developed the concept of the "fight or flight" response to overwhelming danger. He concluded the reactions were initiated in higher centers of the brain and integrated via the sympathetic and parasympathetic nervous systems, stimulating sympathetic responses, with secretion of adrenalin (epinephrine) and inhibition of the parasympathetic system, with corresponding decreases in gut activity. Epinephrine prepared the animal to engage in combat or escape, increasing blood pressure, glucose levels, and delivery of oxygen to muscles and the heart. Inhibition of the parasympathetic system led to decreases in splanchnic (gut) activity—dry mouth, reduced blood flow, and inhibition of gastric secretion and peristalsis. These primitive responses have been observed in both animals and man. Cannon recognized the importance of the human cerebral cortex to integrate the physiologic and emotional responses, and subsequent investigators identified the adrenal gland as the source of epinephrine and related compounds. More recently, unique cells in the brain's temporal cortex—from the Greek "amygdala" because of their almond shape—have been found crucial to responses to threat. These sites are associated with fear, rage, and anxiety. Lesions of the amygdala blunt responses to danger in man or animals.

The study of fear has been a fertile topic for neurophysiologists and psychiatrists for a century. Fear and anxiety have been characterized as adverse reactions to threat, with intense negative feelings and bodily manifestations. Fear denotes dread of impending disaster and the urge to defend oneself or flee, as Cannon deduced. Anxiety is a sense of foreboding, especially if escape or rescue is not likely.

This research has helped explain man's response to danger. Faced with overwhelming threat and potential death, individuals become dreadful, with even greater anxiety. Severe or repetitive episodes may produce PTSD, a response identified in thousands of VN veterans. By 1970, military physicians had identified "neuropsychiatric" problems as the cause of 175,000 days of lost duty, exceeding those lost from malaria, hepatitis, and other medical problems. The war had a profound psychological impact, although identification of PTSD was years in the future. I would soon read an insightful report by an Army psychiatrist that identified soldiers' responses to war and a prelude to the identification of PTSD.

As we cowered in the bunker, I thought of Bac Lieu's residents—crouching in grass shacks or clapboard dwellings, facing attack with no protection. I could imagine the injuries and death. Butchery.

Weapons manuals classify the 75 mm recoilless rifle as a direct-fire anti-armor weapon. But the VC didn't read the books and used these "pack-howitzers" as artillery pieces, firing them at near maximum ranges over flat trajectories. They were far more destructive than mortars. Bac Lieu was being attacked by artillery! Most of the 75s the VC employed were of Chinese origin, although they used captured weapons from the United States, ARVN, and Korea.

The phone in the bunker was inoperable and communication lines had been disrupted. Officers yelled to other bunkers, asking of injuries. Surely, a third attack on the compound would lead to casualties. To our right a huge fire blazed. It wasn't clear if the fire was the motor pool or ammo dump.

The action finally ceased, and the all-clear signal was sounded. Don and I ran to the CP bunker where the colonel and his staff were directing artillery and lightning bugs. The location of the recoilless rifles was known, as a ranger patrol had seen the flashes. The patrol prepared to advance but were told to wait until the end of the 105s' barrage. Lightning bugs were quickly on target and received heavy machine gun fire.

The VC had cleverly established a decoy. They set up automatic weapons in one position, drawing the choppers' attention. The aircraft expended their ammunition and returned to the field to refuel and rearm, as VC attacked from another site.

Standing outside the bunker, we watched flames from the ARVN prison. The captured ammo had indeed sustained a direct hit. Four prisoners were killed in the fire. The lightning bug's tracers were visible as it made passes over the enemy. No Americans had been injured, although several rounds hit the compound and at least one hooch was destroyed. We ran to the hospital to view a catastrophic scene.

The ER was organized confusion. Stretchers and patients were everywhere. VN nurses were bandaging patients and starting IVs. Don, Bill Harris, and Charlie tended wounds, triaged victims, and performed cutdowns for IV access. The most severely injured lay on four tables—all with massive chest wounds. Another dozen with various wounds reposed on the floor and holding area. A 10-year-old girl was carried in by her father; both legs had been blown off above the knee and her back was laid open with a myriad of wounds. We transferred her and two of the chest wounds to surgery, as another chest-abdominal wound entered. Despite fluids and blood donated by Don and Sgt. Hale, the little girl expired within an hour.

For the next eight hours we treated approximately 45 wounded with nine deaths. The number of critically injured patients seemed higher for this attack. Less serious patients were treated and sent home. Several were killed outright in their homes and never reached the hospital.

Charlie, Bill, and I alternated scrubbing with Vinh on the major surgeries, working the ER and fluoroscoping others. Don and the corpsmen supervised the ER and arranged blood donors. Mariana, Joan, Mrs. Vinh, and Pat covered the postoperative areas. Sgt. Hale was scrub nurse, assistant, and morale officer. He said several rounds landed downtown.

"Hell," Hale drawled, "One of the goddamned things even hit the whore house … busted down the front door and almost knocked out the busiest bed in town. The boys will have to find another place to 'clap-out' for a while. That'll serve old Mamason for raising her prices."

We learned a girl in the whore house had been killed, although she was not plying her trade at the time. Her death provided some macabre humor. We concluded bombing a brothel with murder of a popular hostess was a heinous act of war; nay, an escalation and atrocity. What indeed is a more neutral haven than a brothel? Like the Red Cross, it is international and nonsectarian.

"A round in the whore house" and another incident afforded comic relief during a long, painful night. An old drunk was knocked down by a cyclo transporting a patient to the ER. He was not seriously hurt but staggered into the ER. Charlie examined him, dabbed some mercurochrome on the goose egg atop his head, and sent him out. However, each time a new patient arrived, the old man would stumble in and be examined, treated, and discharged. This scenario was repeated several times until he fell asleep on the ER steps.

Time melted away. Soon it was 6:30 a.m. We walked to the compound and treated the Vinhs to eggs, pancakes, and coffee—lots of coffee. After breakfast I wandered around the compound, inspecting the damage, including a hooch a few feet from ours. I also saw the crater of a round near our bunker, the exact site of a hit three months ago. I viewed the remains of the prison's arms cache, several charred bodies, a dud by the back gate, and damage to the motor pool. Several shells landed behind the hospital in the ARVN housing areas—one knocked a hole in the same house where four were killed in February. That afternoon we drove downtown and inspected the whore house. A shell had entered the establishment's front door. Another exploded 20 yards away, destroying a gas station. Two projectiles hit a school, and a shell exploded in front of Dr. Tot's house as a second demolished a shack behind her house—killing one. All ordnance exploded within a radius of 400 meters of the MACV compound and Gen. Minh's house. A round entered the General's bedroom window, but his family were in the basement.

The VC had good aim. They were closer, with better range for the 75s and improved accuracy. Two weapons fired simultaneously from the same position.

The death toll exceeded 30—people killed in town were added to hospital statistics, as well as those who later died. The VC didn't escape unscathed. Gunships caught eight motorized sampans leaving the firing zone, all of which were destroyed, with many secondary explosions. Typically, when patrols visited the scene, no trace of bodies or weapons could be found except empty casings. Col. Gibson grimly reported, "VC use men to defend their weapons; we use weapons to defend our men." A different set of values.

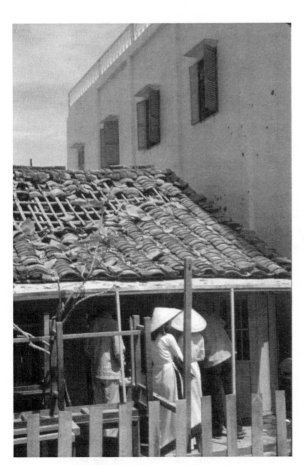

A round in the whore house.

As Bac Lieu was attacked, Vi

Thanh and Vinh Long were also shelled. Luckily no Americans were killed, but the three attacks were synchronized.

Jim arrived on the morning 'bou and didn't learn of the attack until he saw the destroyed hooch next to his. Similarly, a shocked Dr. Homay returned from a visit to the Iranian hospital in Ben Tre. We continued mop-up operations of those injured during the attack. At noon we took a siesta, napping until 2:00 p.m.

Col. Maddox visited the hospital that afternoon, walking from ward to ward, expressing regrets and wishing victims a speedy recovery. Later, a party was held for him, as he would soon leave Bac Lieu for assignment in Germany. The colonel was late. His brother, an Air Force pilot, had been shot down over Hanoi; the news dampened the festivities.

Artillery fired steadily until 11:30 p.m., when the 105s suddenly went silent: a 24-hour truce for Buddha's birthday.

The hospital was closed, but we rounded on the injured. Some patients on Ward 4 had left, fearful of another attack. Other wards remained crowded. Amazingly, those with chest injuries were still alive. The family took the scalped woman home to die. Throughout her ordeal she never complained. Her face haunted me.

Rain and wind attacked with unexpected suddenness, drenching workmen repairing damaged hooches and bunkers.

Aided by the cease fire, the VC moved openly without impediment. A VC regiment (three battalions—nearly 1,500 individuals) was sighted in 50 motorized sampans near Vinh Chau. FAC aircraft were dispatched but could only observe. Whether the VC were regrouping or staging for a future attack was not known, but they used the opportunity for unmolested travel. I thought to myself, "They attacked on the eve of a truce, then took advantage of the cease fire to transport fighters at will; a brazen situation."

Rain swept from the sea, blowing through our hooch as I typed. I was listening to a Brahms piano concerto. How strange! The truce would end at midnight and we would again be at war. A military operation was scheduled for the morning: ARVN would attack the VC, to be followed by another VC strike. Thus, the mayhem proceeded, without pause, an ongoing dance of death. Neither side had a clear advantage, and negotiations were delayed or aborted because of politicians' fear of losing face.

Bac Lieu inhabitants, predominantly simple farmers, bore the fighting's onslaught, caught in the crossfire. Rural life had changed little over a century. But war produced unbelievable suffering, and exposed the government's failure of public health programs, aid to the economy, and education. The VC seized on these weaknesses and dominated peasant life, particularly in the delta.

The following day the hospital resumed a normal status and clinics swelled to preattack levels. Ward patients reentered after days of absence. An elderly man with a chest wound expired, but most of the injured were recovering. Man is resilient.

Capt. Jim Singleton of G2 (intelligence) told us the VC would probably shell Bac Lieu again within a few days. The news was disquieting as his source had predicted the earlier attacks. Everyone was uneasy. One officer remarked, "I feel like a fish in a barrel." The looming crater beside Jim's hooch was a reminder of the

VC's capabilities and our vulnerability. Don and I inspected our bunker. Despite recent repairs, several ceiling planks had caved and many sandbags were splitting. I replaced items in the bunker's medical kit.

There were no light ships that evening, although the moon illuminated a row of clouds to the north. The artillery seemed especially loud. The ground was soggy from a thunderstorm, and the mood was fearful. Several officers maintained a vigil in the club until 3:00 a.m. The EMs were also on edge. After one unusually loud artillery round, several ran to their bunkers. The VC did not strike.

A large ARVN operation near Rach Gia was held. Aircraft dropped tons of ordnance on VC positions, followed by deployment of troops. But the effort was unsuccessful, and few VC were found, another expensive failure.

Vinh operated on a man with TB peritonitis, a rare disease in the States. My views of the prevalence of diseases had changed dramatically since my arrival. Adult clinic typically provided two or three new TB patients, several pneumonias, a variety of parasite infestations, and one or two patients with typhoid or cholera, plus miscellaneous disorders including leprosy or tetanus. To encounter this array of pathology in the United States would require years. The experience was medically fascinating but highlighted the immensity of our task and the plight of delta citizens.

We developed a disaster plan, outlining duties of MACV and USAID personnel in a future attack. Dr. Vinh had workers clear brush and trees behind the hospital for a helicopter landing site. If the airfield were hit or the bridge damaged, a pad would be needed to evacuate casualties.

At least 20 officers took their flak jackets to the evening movie, a silly comedy (*Not With My Wife You Don't*). The precaution was unnecessary, but the movie eased tensions.

In the morning a Caterpillar grader prepared the hospital landing pad as we discussed emergency plans. After an attack, people flock to emergency and triage areas, adding to the confusion and hampering care. MILPHAP medics and hospital workers were assigned to maintain order.

Several motorized sampans were seen near Gia Rai, although no subsequent VC activity was reported.

More rain. The interpreters' *áo dàis* were covered with mud as they walked the rutted street from the center of town after siesta. "Nhieu bun [much mud]," remarked Co Phung.

An ARVN operation was unsuccessful but led to the rescue of two prisoners. A province chief had been captured three years ago. The other was an RD worker, a prisoner for several months. They were held deep in the U Minh forest, along with 80 others, including two Americans. Their meager diet was fish and salted rice, plus occasional vegetables. An opportunity allowed them to strike a guard with a board and flee into the forest where they were rescued by ARVN troops. Another prisoner escaped but was killed by a VC patrol.

The evening's H&I bombardment was intense. Jim and I maintained another graveyard vigil in the officers' club. It is amazing what one will discuss to keep awake. We ultimately retired to our hooches, but the artillery barrage continued until dawn.

I awoke to the sound of another loud noise—thunder, marking the beginning of the VC summer, or monsoon, offensive. General Minh warned the VC would attack district and province capitals with greater intensity.

The compound became the scene of security preparations, both personal and collective. Weapons were cleaned, helmets and ammo belts made ready as bunkers checked for machine guns, supplies, phones, and stretchers. Bac Lieu was on Yellow Alert, the maximum-security threat. The airstrip teemed with gunships, CH47 Chinooks, and giant CH54A Sikorsky flying cranes, as well as Caribous, G123s, and the little L19 FAC planes. Emergency military supplies and medical items were unloaded. Aircraft circled the field throughout the day, waiting to land single file on the short runway. ARVN soldiers arrived for deployment as others unloaded howitzer shells, small arms ammo, and the countless items to fight a war. The U.S. involvement in VN was a logistical marvel, just as the victory of World War II relied upon America's "Arsenal of Democracy."

The USAID nurses were confined to their home. MACV bunkers were now manned by an enlisted man, armed with machine guns and grenade launchers.

Despite rain, wind, and mud, EMs stood guard in the damp bunkers throughout the night. There were reports of VC attacks north of the city, but no other action. Jim and I remained in the officers' club until 5:00 a.m. The "Condition Yellow" status persisted.

The weather cooled, bringing additional rain and "nhieu bun" (much mud), which stuck to boots, trousers, and mats. The VN were less bothered, removing their sandals to wash their feet in a convenient puddle before entering a building.

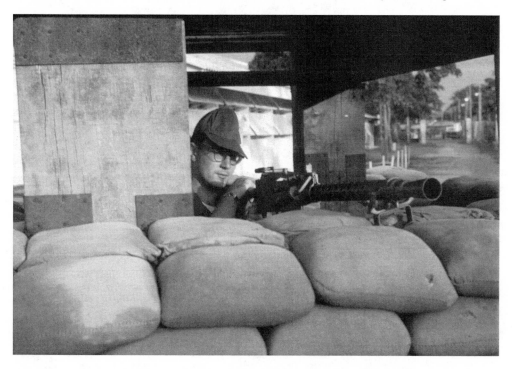

Guard on bunker duty near back gate of MACV compound.

As usual, VC intelligence was excellent and waited for us to relax our guard before another attack. Time favored the enemy. The ARVN division's birthday was June 1, and we anticipated a few surprise gifts. The atmosphere was tense.

Several historians have observed the VC gladly sacrificed men and time to gain military advantage, a practice akin to that documented by Rudyard Kipling of fighting in India a century earlier. The VC picked their battles and waited. The Americans were in a hurry, not the VC.

Because of heightened security, we were forced to examine patients at the back gate during night call. On one visit I saw a woman with pneumonia whose chest was covered with cup marks. Her neck and abdomen bore numerous pinch marks. She had visited the "dong y si" (Chinese doctor). These quacks were also known as "thay bua or thay phap." She asked to come to the hospital, but her husband had faith in the "dong y si." Vinh remarked, "Husband is king, wife is servile in Vietnam." The husband ultimately lost faith in the medicine man and allowed her to see the American Bac Si.

May 30, Memorial Day: The compound observed the holiday, but the hospital was open. I saw a mother and son who had been shot in their sampan by a chopper. Both sustained head wounds. Vinh and Bill Harris operated.

My OB friends at the LA County Hospital sent me a fetoscope. Pat demonstrated the device to the midwives to hear a baby's heartbeat. They had been using an ancient tube-like structure that resembled the stethoscope invented by Laennec 200 years ago. The fetoscope is like a standard stethoscope but has a metal strap over the examiner's head to enhance hearing by bone conduction. The midwives giggled and squirmed like schoolgirls as they took turns listening to an obliging woman.

Although it rained early, the wind cleared the sky by 11:00 a.m., producing a steamy, humid environment. After a noon siesta, I awoke drenched in perspiration.

The Yellow Alert was lifted but we remained on "Condition Gray," a somewhat lower level of readiness.

Chapter Sources

N. Bernard. *Yersin, Pionnier-Savant-Explorateur.* Paris: Editions du Colombler, 1955.

Jack E. Moseley. "Travels of Alexandre Yersin: Letters of a Pastorian in Indochina, 1890–1894." *Perspectives in Biology and Medicine* 24, no. 4 (1981): 607–18.

J. C. Rosenberg. "Doctors Afield: Alexandre Yersin." *New England Journal of Medicine* 278, no. 5 (1968): 261–63.

William Woodruff, MD. Obituary. *JAMA* 286, no. 17 (2001): 2170.

Frederic Pages, M. Faulde, E. Orlandi-Pradines, et al. "The Past and Present Threat of Vector-Borne Diseases in Deployed Troops." *Clinical Microbiology and Infection* 16, no. 3 (2010): 209–24.

Steven J. Berman and William D. Kundin. "Scrub Typhus in South Vietnam: A Study of 87 Cases." *Annals of Internal Medicine* 79, no. 1 (1973): 26–30.

O'Neill Barrett, Jr., and Fred R. Stark. "Rickettsial Diseases and Leptospirosis." Chapter 7 in *Internal Medicine in Vietnam, Vol. II: General Medicine and Infectious Diseases.* Edited by Andre J. Ognibene and O'Neill Barrett, Jr., Washington, D.C.: U.S. Government Printing Office, 1982.

John J. Deller. "Fever of Undetermined Origin." Chapter 4, Part II in *Internal Medicine in Vietnam, Vol. II: General Medicine and Infectious Diseases.* Edited by Andre J. Ognibene and O'Neill Barrett, Jr., Washington, D.C.: U.S. Government Printing Office, 1982.

Merlin L. Brubaker, Chapman H. Binford, and John R. Trautman. "Occurrence of Leprosy in U.S. Veterans After Service in Endemic Areas Abroad." *Public Health Reports* 84, no. 12 (1969): 1051–8.

E. V. Hulse. "The Nature of Biblical 'Leprosy' and the Use of Alternative Medical Terms in Modern Translation of the Bible." *Palestine Exploration Quarterly* 107, no. 2 (1975): 87–105.

Tran Hau Khang, Ngo Mihn Thao, and Le Huu Doanh. "Epidemiology of Leprosy in Vietnam and the Effectiveness of Multidrug Therapy (MDT) in the Management of the Disease." *Current Topics in Neglected Tropical Diseases* (2019).

Frank E. Medford. "Leprosy in Vietnam Veterans." *Archives of Internal Medicine* 134, no. 2 (1974): 373.

Nhiem Nguyen, Thang Tat Nguyen, Hai Hong Phan, et al. "Leprosy: Ongoing Medical and Social Struggle in Vietnam." *Journal of Cutaneous Medicine and Surgery* 12, no. 4 (2006): 147–54.

P. K. Russell and A. J. Ognibene. "Arborviruses." Chapter 5 in *Internal Medicine in Vietnam, Vol. II: General Medicine and Infectious Diseases.* Edited by Andre J. Ognibene and O'Neill Barrett, Jr., Washington, D.C.: U.S. Government Printing Office, 1982.

Robert V. Gibbons, Matthew Streitz, Tatyana Babina, et al. "Dengue and U.S. Military Operations From the Spanish-American War Through Today." *Emerging Infectious Diseases* 18, no. 4 (2012): 623–30.

Matthew S. Goldberg. "Death and Injury Rates of U.S. Military Personnel in Iraq." *Military Medicine* 175, no. 4 (2010): 220–26.

Spurgeon Neel. "Health of the Command." Chapter 2 in *Medical Support of the U.S. Army in Vietnam 1965–1970.* Washington, D.C.: U.S. Government Printing Office, 1973.

_____. "Care of the Wounded." Chapter 3 in *Medical Support of the U.S. Army in Vietnam 1965–1970.* Washington, D.C.: U.S. Government Printing Office, 1973.

Walter B. Cannon. *Bodily Changes in Pain, Hunger, Fear and Rage.* New York: Appleton, 1922.

Daniel H. Funkenstein. "The Physiology of Fear and Anger." *Scientific American* 192, no. 5 (1955): 74–81.

Orion P. Keller, Robert C. Hurt, Kerry J. Ressler, et al. "The Physiology of Fear: Reconceptualizing the Role of the Central Amygdala in Fear Learning." *Physiology* 30, no. 5 (2015): 389–401.

Joseph LeDoux. "Fear and the Brain: Where Have We Been and Where Are We Going?" *Biological Psychiatry* 44, no. 12 (1998): 1229–38.

Ralph Adolphus. "The Biology of Fear." *Current Biology* 23, no. 2 (2013): R79–R93.

A. Ohman. "Fear and Anxiety." Chapter 44 in *Handbook of Emotions.* Edited by M. Lewis, J. M. Haviland-Jones, and L. F. Barrett. New York: Guilford Press, 2008.

11

June

Drinking Songs, VD, and Dalat

Col. Maddox completed his tour as commander of the MACV advisory team. Officers and enlisted personnel lined the runway to pay their respects as Maddox made a few final remarks then walked onto the Caribou, bound for Germany. The new senior officer held a briefing that afternoon. He was of medium height, with sharply chiseled features and rapid-fire speech, a picture of military confidence. A man of the book, he emphasized unprofessional behavior would not be tolerated. This was his second VN tour. I was unable to gain an impression of our new commander, but events soon revealed clues to his emotions.

Mariana made her weekly pilgrimage to the Chieu Hoi repatriation center, returning with a patient. An inmate had an argument with his wife, claiming she insulted him in front of his comrades. To spite his wife and regain "face," he cut off a finger. This act was dramatic, but senseless from a Western perspective. Dr. Vinh repaired the stump this afternoon.

My evening schedule had evolved. After typing and bereft of sleep, I'd retire to the officers' club until the wee hours in the air-conditioned room. An added benefit was muffling of the artillery sounds. Sitting alone or with a "short-timer," I'd try to read; but fear of an attack remained, and it was difficult to concentrate. The few remaining in the club drank themselves into a daze. I would ultimately return to my hooch for two or three hours of rest.

We visited the dispensary at Gia Rai, taking a sampan for the final 3 km. The wooden watercraft were equipped with a long shaft outboard motor to position the propeller just below the water's surface, as depth was only two or three feet. The bows were adorned with eyes to guide the tiny vessels and protect them from evil spirits. We sat on our haunches on the boat's flat bottom as we passed half-empty rice paddies and small hamlets. Some banks were barren, others lined with trees, blocking the view. These areas were prime sites for ambushes, and our guards were uneasy during these passages. Some canal scenes resembled a bucolic picture postcard.

The Gia Rai clinic had been renovated, resupplied, and restaffed. The workers were eager to show us the facilities but told us they lived in constant fear of assassination or attack. I tried to imagine survival under such constant threat. Gia Rai remained unsecure and our major source of VC-induced trauma.

131

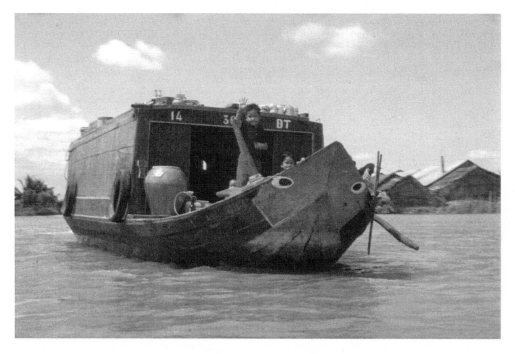

Sampan with "eyes" on local canal.

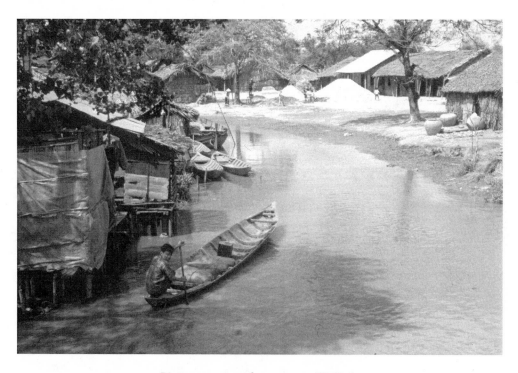

Picturesque canal scene near Gia Rai.

Hospital activity was slow. The surgery workers dried moldy scrub suits and surgical gowns in the sun, the first day without rain for more than a week.

Co Phung invited us to her house for ice cream and pointed out the sandbags in their living room where they hid during attacks. The family had another home downtown, but it had been bombed three times.

Don Robinson presided over a MILPHAP promotion ceremony for Sgt. Hale and Spc. Manzo. We retired to the NCO club for congratulatory drinks. There was considerable celebration in the officers' club. No movie was shown, and serious drinking began earlier than usual. By 8:00 p.m., several inebriated officers were singing. The songs were in poor taste. One version of "Wake the Town" included these verses:

> Strafe the town and kill the people.
> Bomb the schools and churches too.
> Show the kiddies in the playground
> What a napalm run can do.
> Shoot your rockets at the building
> With the red cross on the door;
> Then send in the troops to rape and plunder—
> That's the way to fight the war.

Other songs portrayed the weariness of war, as this rendition of "Take Me Out to the Ball Game":

> Take me off of the Vinh Strike,
> Take me out of the war.
> Write me some orders and send me back,
> I've had enough of the Triple A flak.
> For they shoot, shoot, shoot at my little craft,
> If you send me to Hanoi, I'll scream.
> Oh, it's one, two, three strikes a day,
> On the old yankee team.

Finally, one tune had horrendous overtones:

> Drop a 10 kt from your A4E;
> The only way to win is to escalate.
> We'll engulf them all in a fireball;
> The radiation rate will be simply great.
> All dressed in snowy white, with a squeal of delight,
> You'll pull out at burst height.
> It's seventh heaven …
> So kill the Viet Cong in your A4E
> And never ever ban the bomb.

One might excuse the drunken singers, and perhaps the songs were only satire, tension-relieving gestures. But the drunken men relished in the frightening verses. Several officers were offended and left the club.

The behavior illustrated frustration, disillusionment, and a callous attitude toward the civilian population. Vietnam was the second Asian conflict in less 15 years in which the United States fought a communist force that attacked a sister country from the north. But analogies with the Korean war are few. North and

South Korea were ideologically distinct, and territory south of the 38th parallel was contested. The DMZ was an important demarcation, but Vietnam was also fighting a civil war. Support for the Korean war was strong; nearly 80 percent approved Truman's 1950 military assistance. By 1953 opinion had eroded somewhat, but more than 50 percent of American citizens still supported the war. In contrast, the psychological impact of the Vietnam War was enormous, reflecting the unique nature of the conflict as recorded by scholars. Hochgesang et al. concluded Vietnam differed from prior U.S. wars in at least three ways: The conflict was increasingly unpopular with soldiers as well as the American public. Second, it was the first war to be covered intensely by media, magnifying distrust and lack of government transparency. Finally, these factors influenced soldiers' attitudes in an ever-confusing war. As described earlier, fear and anxiety led to depression, panic attacks, and ultimately, PTSD. Another result was loss of morale and trust in one's comrades and superiors. The average soldier was a teenager and stress his constant companion. Shortly after high school new draftees received eight weeks of training, to arrive in an undeveloped country with a foreign culture. The major concern was to stay alive to date of expected return from overseas (DEROS). The war was confusing. Territory was not sought as in traditional combat and there were no front lines. Disillusionment and hopelessness were fueled by drug and alcohol abuse, which affected many soldiers in some units. In contrast, officers were supposed to be professional soldiers to conduct the war. Tensions developed between EMs and officers. Hostility between the groups boiled over with "fragging," in which an officer was injured or killed by tripping a fragmentation grenade rigged by his men. More than 730 fragging episodes were documented between 1969 and 1975, predominantly in northern I, II, and III Corps. Drug abuse and resentment, justified or not, played a role in many of these events. Most of these crimes were never successfully prosecuted.

Hatred became focused on the Vietnamese citizen. Initially, the North Vietnamese were the enemy, but the VC emerged as a major foe. They were invisible, indistinguishable from civilians who frequently harbored them. No one could be trusted. Ultimately, all Vietnamese were suspect. They were not only foreign but viewed as racially inferior. A variety of terms dehumanized the citizens and made them untrustworthy. Why were we dying to defend their country when they didn't deserve or want our help? The difficulties faced by soldiers of color were amplified. The discrimination they faced was often transferred to hatred of Vietnamese, or their superior officers.

The behavior in the club was not representative of most officers, but it wasn't isolated. MACV advisors experienced a closer relationship with their ARVN counterparts than most soldiers. Nevertheless, the drunken singers displayed hostility, bigotry, frustration, and a lack of trust of the Vietnamese. The songs illustrated the emotional scars and jumbled feelings of many servicemen.

Jim did not hear the serenades. He was on call, struggling to save a pregnant woman with eclampsia (seizures and hypertension). The woman died before morning.

The rains returned, although more gently. The inclement weather brought new casualties—victims of VC booby traps.

Don Robinson received his orders. His DEROS was less than two months away, and he would be discharged on return to the United States. He began his 60-day calendar—a drawing of a nude woman marked in numbered segments. Each day a new patch was tacked onto the body; at 60 days she would be fully clothed.

We awoke to the sound of a squadron of B-52s returning from Cambodia. By 6:00 a.m., a fierce southwesterly wind dropped the temperature and rain blew through the sides of the hooches, soaking our beds. When I stepped outside, the boardwalks were afloat, and a rain gauge measured several inches. We would endure summer monsoon weather for the next few months.

The hospital was quiet as few braved mud and mire to attend morning clinics. When Jim made maternity rounds, most of the midwives were still asleep.

At 5:00 p.m., we were called to the ER to examine a girl of 13 years, "marching" through a Jacksonian seizure (convulsion). Despite massive doses of sedation medications, she continued to seize every few minutes.

Jacksonian seizures begin in one location of the body and "march" to other muscle groups. In the 1860s and 1870s, the famous English neurologist John H. Jackson first described this seizure and identified the area of the brain causing the episode. Neurology in the 19th century was mostly descriptive as little could be done therapeutically. Doctors followed patients until death, then painstakingly examined the brain and spinal cord to correlate anatomy with antemortem symptoms. We ultimately controlled her seizures and admitted her.

Life for Bac Lieu's poor was never easy, but sometimes their burden was excessively cruel, as a hard luck day in clinic confirmed. In addition to the usual, "dau bungs" (aches), pneumonias, and worms, the first unhappy tale involved a Cambodian woman. She had contracted trachoma (a bacterial infection of the eye) as a youth and was completely blind, although today's complaint involved her pet cat. This morning she couldn't find the animal and heard soldiers outside her hut discussing their evening supper. They found her cat and proceeded to kill and cook the animal. Cats, dogs, rats, and other animals were considered appropriate food in rural areas, although many people kept pets. When she learned of her cat's fate, she ran outside and verbally attacked the solders, yelling and cursing. They returned her taunts with physical abuse, which led to her hospital visit for multiple bruises and lacerations.

The second tale of woe was a VC's wife who requested admission. Her husband had deserted her, and she and her child bartered to eke out a meager existence. A week earlier a gunship cornered a group of insurgents in an adjoining hut, firing rockets and machine guns. The missiles missed the VC's hut but burned her shack and destroyed her belongings. I learned the story from the interpreter as I examined the woman. She had pneumonia, and I admitted her to the hospital. We could treat her lung infection, but her problems were only delayed. When discharged, she and her child had no place to live or source of food. Perhaps the Red Cross had solved the problems at the refugee center where she could seek shelter—although I doubted it.

Late-night drinkers kept the bar open most nights. Among the group was a major, who was depressed and a frequent night owl. He drank heavily, blunting his depression. He was a short-timer, and I could only speculate his future. Alcohol or drugs are frequent companions of mental illnesses, used to blunt symptoms.

The 1988 Veterans Readjustment Study estimated more than 250,000 Veterans suffered from PTSD, and up to 30 percent of returning veterans would experience a lifetime rate of PTSD. There was a very strong association between PTSD and combat exposure, but even those who did not see battle were affected. Depression, homelessness, substance abuse,

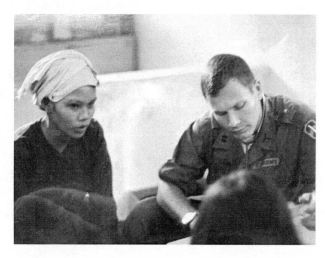
Homeless VC woman and author.

suicide, and other disorders plagued veterans for decades. Because of the public's disfavor of the war, men also faced rejection and discrimination, further alienating them from society, and hampering identification and treatment. Although PTSD had been the subject of psychiatric literature for years, it was not officially identified by the American Psychiatric Association until 1987. The findings of the Veterans Readjustment Study have been challenged and the subject of multiple scientific publications, but the seriousness of the problem has not been disputed, nor its destruction of so many lives. More current estimates of the lifetime prevalence of PTSD among veterans are approximately 18 percent, with ongoing psychiatric problems in up to 9 percent. VN studies increased awareness of PTSD for the Iraq and Afghanistan conflicts, as well as PTSD resulting from civilian trauma.

For years I experienced nightmares, flashbacks, difficulty concentrating, and lack of intimacy and ability to form close friendships, typical features of mild PTSD. I did not discuss my experiences in Vietnam and avoided items that intensified VN memories, such as movies, books, and my diary. I sought psychiatric support for an interval, but my symptoms were minor compared to those who struggled with mental health problems for decades.

Charlie returned from his Hawaii R&R, replete with flowered shirts, suntan, and fond memories of ice cream. But the trip alerted him to the fury of antiwar sentiments in the United States. Meanwhile, Secretary McNamara commissioned the Vietnam Study Task Force, subsequently termed the Pentagon Papers, which Daniel Ellsberg leaked to the press in 1971. The documents exposed the futility of the war as well as the government's duplicity.

The loop clinic placed more than 30 IUDs one morning. Patients came from as far away as Ca May, Soc Trang, and Can Tho. News of the "baby prevention clinic" had spread throughout the delta. Two women brought their IUDs in neatly packaged newspapers. The devices had become dislodged, and the women wanted them reinserted. They were surprised when the midwives discarded the used IUDs, as they had no concept of sterility or disposable equipment. USAID officials in Can Tho warned me the MOH had learned of the clinic and might order closure of the project. Jim asked the head midwife to be more discreet in broadcasting news of the clinic.

Jim's liberal opinions sometimes led to conflict. In the club one evening, Jim and an officer tangled over political and religious topics. Following an exchange that featured Martin Luther King, the man called Jim "one of those left-wing extremists." Jim bristled, but continued his discourse, suggesting Christ was probably the first proponent of civil disobedience. After a moment of reflection, the young lieutenant's eyes flashed as he exclaimed, "Yes, but look what happened to him!" The remark broke up the discussion and the respective speakers retreated to the safety of their supporters.

As we walked to the latrine the next morning, we were greeted by a sign: *Water Pump Broken—Use EM latrine*. Grudgingly, we went to the EM facility. The cause of the plumbing fiasco soon became clear. The new commanding officer ordered all jeeps to be washed daily. The VN workers decided they could use water from the officers' latrine to save a trip downtown where there was a high-pressure water line. The limited supply of potable water was quickly expended, the pump overheated and failed. The colonel's compulsive behavior precipitated the incident; a trait I would better understand in the coming months.

Care of patients was guided by clinical judgment and our meager laboratory facilities, but an episode in clinic made me question my competence. I examined an elderly woman I had seen two months earlier for a bloody cough (hemoptysis). At the first visit, I wrote an order for a TB sputum analysis, X-ray, and a TB skin test, together with cough syrup. She was told to return in a week. The woman had the skin test, gave the sputum sample, and collected the cough syrup, but didn't have the X-ray or return, despite cough, fatigue, and fever. She went to the local spiritualist and was "cupped." I checked the TB sputum results and read the one-word answer in capital letters: *YES!* She had advanced TB and I admitted her to the female ward. I should have done so initially but believed she would heed my instructions. Ignorance and folk remedies were powerful influences.

Tuberculosis (TB), the white plague or phthisis, has affected civilization since the dawn of time. Hippocrates and Galen described many of its symptoms, and the organism has killed peasants and kings for millennia. In the latter part of the 19th century several therapies were developed, including collapse of the upper lobes to "rest the lungs" and allow cure. The brutal methods had some favorable effect, although the mechanism was unknown at the time. A current explanation for their partial success is they reduced ventilation to the upper lung areas, which are richer in oxygen due to regional distribution of ventilation and perfusion of blood. The TB bacillus prospers in an oxygen rich area—hence, the upper lobes are the most frequent sites of TB. Despite these barbaric procedures, there was no effective treatment. Doctors advocated a move to warmer climes—as did the gambler-dentist Doc Holliday who ventured to Arizona for his famous Tombstone liaison with Wyatt Earp. Somewhat later the concept of bed rest and nutritious food led to the sanitarium movement. The disease was occasionally contained, but not cured. In 1884, the eminent microbiologist Robert Koch identified the tubercle bacillus, for which he

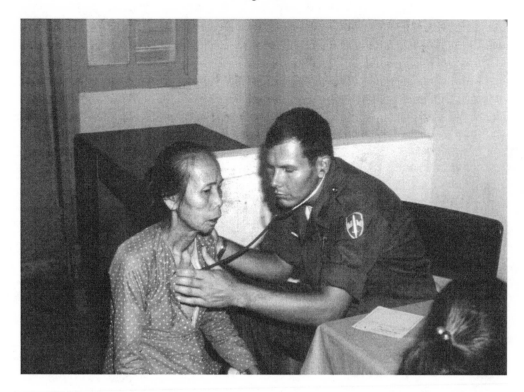

TB patient and author in clinic—note lack of face masks.

received the Nobel prize. Early in the 20th century the French physicians Calmette and Guerin developed the BCG vaccine. But effective treatment awaited the development of the antibiotic streptomycin in the 1940s. Other drugs soon followed, as it quickly became apparent the organism develops resistance to a single drug. By the 1960s, "triple drug therapy" was standard and effective. Highly resistant strains have now emerged, with a world-wide resurgence of the disease and search for new antimicrobials.

Awakening to a dull migraine, I trudged to the Phan Dinh Phung hospital to hold clinic. Suddenly, a PFC ran to the door and shouted Steve needed help. I ran to an EM hooch where Steve was giving mouth to mouth resuscitation to a prostrate soldier. The story was garbled, but the man became short of breath after drinking. He developed stridor, spasm of the larynx, and passed out. The episode was likely an anaphylactic attack. We gave him epinephrine, obtained a stretcher, and within minutes he was on the hospital operating table for a tracheostomy. As we operated, Stoney called for a dust off to evac him. The chopper landed in the new helipad behind the hospital, raising clouds of dust. Once its human cargo had been loaded, the dust off was aloft, flying north.

VC attacked another local outpost. A watch tower sustained a direct hit, killing eight ARVN soldiers. Air support was called from Can Tho, and Spooky threw lead at the VC with its multiple weapons. Spooky, or "Puff the Magic Dragon," of the Peter, Paul and Mary song, was an amazing contraption. I read a description of Spooky by John Steinbeck in the *Chicago Tribune*:

It is a C-47, that old Douglas two-motor ship that has been the workhorse of the world since early in WWII. I don't know who designed puff, but whoever did had imagination. It is armed with three six-barreled gatling guns. In one-fourth of a turn, these fixed guns fine-tooth an area bigger than a foot-ball field, and so completely that not even a tuft of crab-grass would remain alive. The ships, some of them, are in the air every area at night and all night. If a call for help comes, they can be there in a very short time.

Such a call came the next night. At such times I was glad old Puff, or whatever the hell one called it, was up there. But it was a frightful weapon and killed several VC that evening.

The VC distributed leaflets threatening to attack Bac Lieu. In response to such threats, hospital volume fell. Fearing an attack, patients left the wards, despite ongoing illness. Most warnings were not acted upon. Terror is real, if only a threat.

Unhappy rumors of the loop clinic proved to be correct. Dr. Douglas wrote: "'Population control' had been discussed at the MOH which concluded no population explosion exits in VN. Furthermore, VN law prohibits birth control. The MOH suggested any activity be limited to individual family planning via private organizations—outside the VN government."

We were livid and Jim fumed over the MOH disregard of people's welfare. If population were assessed by land area, the number of Vietnam's citizens was not excessive. But peasant women were forced to bear eight or more children for two or three to reach adulthood, and they couldn't afford to feed the ones they bore. The result was malnourished, chronically ill peasants. USAID spent millions to support the MOH but could not dictate policy. We were angry, but on reflection Jim concluded we had not been ordered to stop the clinic and were in compliance with their mandate of private family planning. We vowed to quietly continue our efforts. The saga of the birth control clinic was just beginning.

I learned the enlisted man evacuated with the airway problem had improved and was transferred to Vung Tau for recuperation. Steve's fast action saved the man's life.

Vinh, Charlie, and I operated on a man with a neck wound. The trauma was weeks old but led to a baseball-sized carotid artery aneurysm. An aneurysm is a balloon-like defect of a blood vessel, usually an artery, from trauma or congenital condition. The term "aneurysm" is derived from the Greek for "dilation." The weakened area is prone to burst with devastating consequences. The carotid arteries supply blood to the brain and rupture could be fatal or cause a massive stroke.

The large, pulsating mass was an ominous reminder that disaster could befall any error during surgery. We tried to persuade Dr. Vinh to send the patient to Can Tho, which had vascular surgery expertise—but "Steel Nerves" Vinh insisted he would proceed. All went well initially, but the aneurysm suddenly burst. Blood spewed everywhere, covering surgical drapes, gowns, and our faces. Fortunately, Vinh had isolated the artery proximal to the defect and was able to clamp the vessel and stem the bleeding. The man was young, so occluding one of the arteries feeding his brain did not cause a stroke, because of collateral circulation. The remainder of the surgery was uneventful. Once again, Vinh demonstrated his surgical prowess and his fearlessness. Charlie and I rolled our eyes as Vinh calmly sutured the wound.

ARVN troops were on Yellow Alert and Bac Lieu off limits. Gen. Minh had deployed more than 2,000 troops around the city. Rumors of VC activity was widely circulated, and the night's sky was illuminated by flare ships, with Spooky awaiting duty.

The lethal aircraft did not have long to wait. An ARVN unit was hit near the city. The light ship illuminated the area and Spooky began firing its gatling guns. Hearing the melee, we could also see the tracers. A tracer is every fifth bullet and illuminates the line of fire. The stream of red appeared constant, as several of Spooky's guns were firing simultaneously. Thousands of rounds of ammo were expended within minutes. What an awesome killing machine!

In addition to Spooky's action, additional battles were joined. Three VC platoons were surprised by an ARVN patrol, and a fierce fight ensued. The delta war was hot.

During evening vigils in the club or Jim's hooch, we chatted for hours to pass the time and ease the fearful sounds of the artillery. Jim was a wise counsel, and our discussions were wide ranging: medicine, philosophy, literature, and life after Vietnam. He was thrilled with research and fascinated with pathophysiology—the quest to understand the mechanisms of disease. I had no hunger to return to Ob-Gyn and pondered my post–Vietnam career. Jim reminded me the similarities of our Vietnam tasks and the treatment of the underserved in the United States. He said, "Dick, you can marry clinical service and an academic career—medical schools are usually based in public hospitals, a perfect combination."

Jim returned to Vung Tau for a follow-up of his hepatitis. I assisted Vinh operate on a young Cambodian boy with peritonitis. Instead of a ruptured appendix or typhoid lesion, we found a bowel perforation and were greeted by three 8" ascaris worms wriggling freely in the abdomen. I shook my head in disbelief as we removed the beasts from the operative field.

Ascaris lumbricoides is a roundworm or nematode found in countries with poor hygiene and is possibly the most common parasite in the world. Adult worms can reach a length of 14 inches. Eggs released in feces are ingested with soil-contaminated food. They develop into larvae and penetrate the intestine, migrating to the lungs where they are coughed up and swallowed. Again, in the intestine, larvae mature to adult worms, producing eggs, which are defecated with feces—completing the cycle. *Ascaris* infestation was extremely common in Vietnam, especially among children with repeated bouts. An antiparasitic drug was available but infrequently used because of reinfections. Few Americans were affected by the parasite.

Premier Ky visited Bac Lieu. Police and ARVN cleared city streets and troops were stationed throughout the area. A military band arrived, and city officials lined the street awaiting Ky's arrival, along with curious residents, children, dogs, pigs, and vendors.

A trio of gunships circled the airfield. After establishing security, the choppers landed, offloading Premier Ky and his entourage who boarded awaiting jeeps. Troops saluted as the motorcade passed. The convoy parked at General Minh's headquarters and were greeted by city officials as the band played. In addition to Major General Nguyen Cao Ky, the Premier and Air Vice Marshal, were General Cao Van

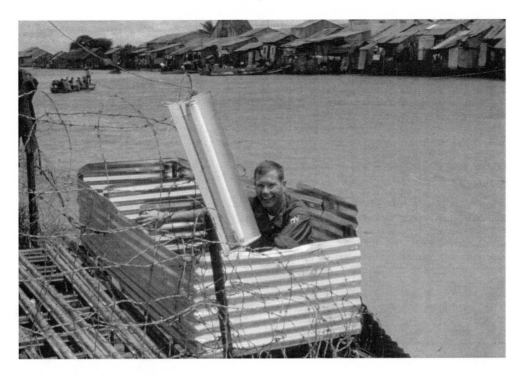

Author sitting in a latrine over a major Bac Lieu canal.

Vien, Chief of the General Staff; Major General Nguyen Duc Thang, Minister of Revolutionary Development; Major General Nguyen Van Minh, Commander in Chief of Region IV; and Brigadier General Desobry, IV Corps Senior Advisor.

Premier Ky was a handsome man of average height, sharp features, and a well-cropped mustache. He wore pressed tropical khakis and a black baseball cap topped with two stars to indicate his rank of major general, plus a silk scarf: a dashing figure.

Gen. Minh gave a welcoming speech, followed by remarks from Ky, who awarded medals to rangers who had distinguished themselves during recent attacks. Five American advisors also received awards. Young girls in their finest *áo dài s* placed leis around the recipients as NBC and VN photographers recorded the event. The party walked across the street for photo ops at a display of captured VC weapons—recoilless rifles, 20 mm cannons, machine guns, mortars, and rifles.

Ky spent the night in Bac Lieu, guarded by Spooky, gunships, and FACs. Thankfully, the 105s were silent, providing a night's rest for the dignitaries as well as those in the compound.

Nguyen Cao Ky (1930–2011) was a pilot and chief of Vietnam's Air Force during the early 1960s. He was involved in the coup that assassinated Diem, followed by election to prime minister, 1965–67. He later served as vice president under his rival, Nguyen Van Thieu. Ky was a provocative, colorful character, married three times and disliked by many for his vanity. He fled Vietnam as the government fell and moved to Southern California. He later returned to Vietnam, urging reconciliation and joint financial ventures. He died in 2011 and is buried in California.

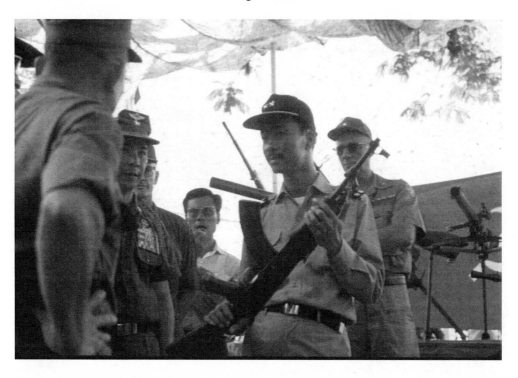

At a display of captured VC weapons: Unknown, Gen. Minh, two unknown officers, Gen. Ky, and Gen. Desobry.

The next morning Premier Ky departed amid a protective shield of gunships. The remainder of the day was quiet, befitting a Sunday.

Vinh held a farewell dinner for Bill Harris. Vinh respected Bill's vegan allegiance by serving a large fruit, termed "sau rieng" in VN—Durian in French. As big as a pineapple, it has a spiny covering. Inside is a sweet mass of semisolid goo—the taste and pervasive odor are overwhelming, although it is a delicacy throughout the Orient. Bill obliged by eating two portions, although I could not tolerate the smelly item.

Dr. William Harris declared his veganism in 1950 and became a popular advocate. A brilliant student, he graduated from the University of California School of Medicine and practiced in California for many years. A pilot and member of Mensa, he wrote and lectured extensively on vegetarianism. He moved to Hawaii, where he cofounded the Vegetarian Society of Hawaii (William Harris, MD, 1930–2015).

Another tragic story awaited me in the ER where a woman squatted with her two-year-old son. The boy had been shot in the arm. The father, an ARVN soldier, was carrying the child near a Ca Mau outpost. He heard gunfire and saw choppers engaging the enemy. The man hurried for protection to his post, shielding his son against his chest. A sniper spotted the pair and fired—the bullet passed through the child's forearm, shattering both bones, and entered the father's left chest, killing him instantly. The boy was rescued by other soldiers. A military burial was held two days later, following which the mother loaded the child and their belongings on a bus to Bac Lieu. As the injury occurred days earlier, the wound was badly infected. The widow would receive a meager allowance from the government.

Military duty included fighting and sometimes legal proceedings. The chapel was the scene of a special court martial of a PFC who was accused of sleeping at his post. The charge was serious, especially during conflict. One found guilty during war was subject to a general court martial and could face a death sentence. But technically we were not at war, although it felt like one. A special court martial could impose a six-month sentence and forfeit salary. The findings would be reviewed at a higher level, subject to modifications.

There were no lawyers, but the officers assigned to defense and prosecution took their responsibilities seriously. Jim was on the evaluation panel. The key issue was if the sergeant of the guard could document the allegation. There were no witnesses except a VN guard. Testimony was taken and cross-examined. Unfortunately, Don and I were called away before the end of the trial, but learned the accused was found guilty. The outcome would be known in a month. Sleeping on guard duty is a serious matter—four days after the incident, the VC shelled the compound.

Bac Lieu remained on high alert.

A new team member arrived on the 'bou: Joe Neal, a second-year medical student from Stanford. A sandy-haired chunky fellow from Modesto, California, he was probably the only medical student to volunteer for the AMA. His enthusiasm was obvious and his tenure memorable. In correspondence to me years later, Joe reflected on his experiences with humility and recalled Jim's comments of the court martial. Although Jim had irreverent views of the military, he was impressed by the professionalism of the trial and the participants.

In addition to Joe, two AMA physicians joined our group: Dr. Jack Redman, a generalist from Albuquerque, and Dr. Merritt W. Stark, a pediatrician from Denver. Dr. Stark's son was a marine serving in Da Nang.

The final exam for midwife students was scheduled but the chief midwife was visiting Can Tho. Jim, a board-certified obstetrician, became the examiner. The questions were difficult, but one struggling applicant came up with a clever response to a query. When pressed for the correct treatment for a very sick mother, the student answered, "I would invite Dr. Jones to see the patient." A flattered but embarrassed Jim gave the enterprising student a passing grade.

More surgery for Dr. Vinh—a radical mastectomy for a nun with breast cancer. I was called that evening multiple times by her anxious colleagues who held a vigil at her bedside.

Our team was honored at the town hall. Local

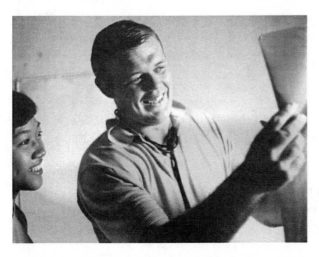

Interpreter Co Tuyet and medical student Joe Neal in clinic.

officials gave speeches, and we were awarded a brass plaque by the city council. Following the festivities, entertainment and food were served at the province chief's home. As usual, cognac was the most popular beverage.

Jim was called to the maternity ward for a moribund postpartum woman. She arrived by sampan from a VC-controlled area. Fearing arrest, her husband did not come. The almost lifeless body was unloaded from a cyclo. Her blood pressure was low; she was in coma and near death. The illness was most likely a postpartum infection. An IV was started and she was given medication to raise the blood pressure. Jim told the distraught family the woman would succumb. Hearing the news, the family asked for the patient be released to die at home or en route. The patient was

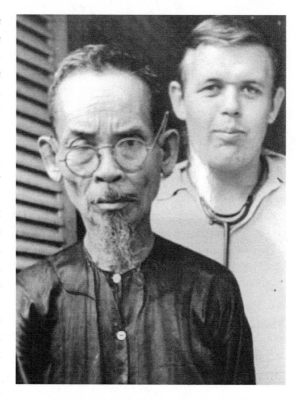

Chinese TB patient and Joe Neal.

again loaded onto a cyclo and the unhappy group departed. The event was typical of many unhappy journeys—a poor family transporting a dying or deceased loved one to a hut for a simple burial. The wails of the patient's mother could be heard above the noise of the cyclo's engine as it traversed the muddy driveway.

The 21st divisional band gave a concert in the EM club. The father of one of our interpreters led the 40-piece group through several marches and popular songs. It reminded me of halftime at a high school basketball game. The concert ended with playing the VN and American anthems.

Steve and I drove to the airport to fly to Can Tho for a military medical update. Our Beechcraft was late because of bad weather that threatened as we boarded. The pilot said he needed to make a stop at Vi Thanh en route. We took off, but were quickly surrounded by clouds as ceiling dropped to less than 300 feet. We descended and circled but couldn't locate the Vi Thanh airstrip. Descending to 100 feet, the pilot saw a canal and followed it until we saw the city. Flying low over canals and tree lines was dangerous—especially near Vi Thanh, site of several recent VC incidents. Luckily, we found the airport, landed, and were quickly aloft to Can Tho. The senior advisor's chopper, which followed us, was less fortunate. They also encountered low ceiling and were forced to fly at low altitude above a canal. Their chopper came under machine gun fire and several rounds hit the craft. Fortunately, no one was injured and the Huey remained air-worthy. The self-sealing capabilities of its fuel tanks prevented a disaster.

The Can Tho medical meeting was not very interesting, but predictable. The topic was VD. Like the poor, venereal disease will always be with us—especially in the military. Some commanders were offended if more than 1–2 percent of their troops became infected. An experiment had been conducted in Can Tho to determine if routine physicals of "local girls," plus weekly injections of penicillin, would lower the soldiers' rate of VD. The Can Tho experiment was a resounding failure—the incidence of VD soared. Multiple factors contributed to the poor results. One was the assumption that inspections and antibiotics would protect if personal hygiene practices such as condoms were abandoned. A zillion units of penicillin will not prevent disease if one has intercourse with a girl who had just slept with an infected individual.

Venereal disease (VD) and drug abuse were rampant among American forces in Vietnam, as in most wars. The incidence of VD was 261 per 1,000 troop strength per year from 1963 to 1970, and VD was the most common medical diagnosis of all diseases. Gonorrhea (GC) accounted for 90 percent of cases. Statistically, more than one in four soldiers developed GC yearly, and many had repeated infections. VD educational programs were largely ineffective, and most servicemen did not use prophylaxis. At that time GC was susceptible to penicillin so patients were treated in clinic, returning the soldier to duty.

When we returned from Can Tho we were pleasantly surprised to learn Dr. Vinh's promise of a Dalat trip had been approved.

Jim performed a radial hysterectomy, a rare procedure in Bac Lieu. The availability of this operation for uterine cancer was crucial, as there was no radiation therapy, and transport to Saigon was difficult, expensive, and dangerous. Although we lived in a war zone, cancer and other "civilian" diseases affected the populace as frequently as elsewhere. Vinh was impressed by Jim's surgical expertise.

Army radio reported the VC sank a navy Swift boat as it cruised a few hundred yards offshore. The enemy used a 75 mm recoilless rifle to disable the 50-foot vessel. No Americans were killed, although there were several injuries. The vessel sank in 25 feet of water and was abandoned. It took two shells from the recoilless rifle to sink the boat, which was pretty good shooting.

Swift boats, or Patrol Craft Fast, were used extensively during the delta war. The aluminum vessels carried a crew of six, including a commanding officer. Boats could achieve speeds of more than 30 knots and were employed for coastal and inland waters. The vessels carried twin 50-caliber machine guns and mortars. John Kerry was a decorated commander of a Swift boat. His service and awards were disputed during the 2004 presidential campaign, although the allegations were later discredited.

Rain and more artillery—the 105 mm guns battered all day, as a VC heavy weapons unit was sighted nearby. Army shotgun planes supported the ARVN artillery. Shotguns were small two-place aircraft with similar missions as FAC, although they usually didn't direct air strikes. Both planes were used for reconnaissance, flew above convoys, and relayed enemy positions. Once the smoke had cleared, the ARVN patrol rescued four prisoners and captured several VC. One of the shotgun aircraft was hit in the wing. Again, self-sealing tanks prevented fire or loss of fuel.

Jim received news that UCSF had approved the surgical refresher program for Vinh. The Bac Si was ecstatic but apprehensive of a visit to "Hoa Ky." It was my task to arrange the trip's logistics with USAID in Saigon.

Alphabet soup was alive and well in government: USAID became CORDS—Civilian Operations for Revolutionary Development and Support. Although USAID remained under civilian control, provincial representatives would report to the MACV colonel, which was a problem for our team.

Charlie initiated the "Bac Lieu Medical School" curriculum as he tutored Joe Neal in clinic. The topic of the day was physical diagnosis. Obliging patients allowed Joe to identify and confirm Charlie's findings. The clinic was a gold mine of pathology. Joe was also given assignments in the medical ward, including patients with TB. Jim took Joe under his wing and tutored him on a variety of topics, including how to examine the abdomen, the gentle, probing skill of the surgeon.

The nurses hosted the team to a chicken dinner, complete with corn on the cob, sweet potatoes, and ice cream from the Phung's store. Midway through the meal, electrical power was lost, leading to candlelight dining. The girls' home was not equipped with a generator and power failures were frequent because of the city's unreliable electricity. Their two-story brick and cement house had an interesting, but sordid, history. The structure was built decades earlier by a wealthy Frenchman, complete with tile floors, exotic woods, high ceilings, and overhead fans, but primitive electrical and plumbing systems. The home featured a 5,000-gallon water tank on the roof and a cistern that had been converted to a bomb shelter. During the Indochina war, the French used the house as an interrogation center for political prisoners. There were numerous stories of torture, atrocities, and acts of violence. Many townspeople believed the dwelling was haunted. USAID acquired the structure from the city and partially refurnished it, but plumbing and electrical issues persisted.

Rain, rain, rain. The boardwalks connecting the hooches were afloat, and adjoining ponds filled with drowned rats, frogs and two green snakes.

We prepared for our Dalat trip. I felt guilty leaving the hospital without physician coverage except for the volunteer physicians and Joe, but Dr. Vinh promised a memorable visit to the mountain retreat.

Our adventure began with a flight to Saigon, where we spent the night at the USAID facility. Early the next morning we boarded a courier aircraft to Dalat. Within an hour our plane descended through thick clouds, circled a wide, lush valley, and landed at Dalat. The airfield was surrounded by pine trees and plantations. A short drive through gentle hills and wooded countryside brought us to the Palace hotel, an impressive three-story cement building atop a hill overlooking a serene lake. The Palace is a classic structure built by the French in the 1920s. We registered and were shown to our chambers, climbing an elegant wooden stairway. Our rooms featured high ceilings, large windows, overhead fans, and large canopied beds with mosquito netting. Bathrooms were fitted with marble, gleaming tile and antique brass fixtures, mammoth bathtubs, and bidets. The hotel has been upgraded since the war and is currently a popular tourist location, with modern conveniences and wisps of prior French elegance.

The weather was refreshingly cool. We changed into sport coats to meet Vinh in the lobby for our drive to the province hospital, where we were introduced to two of his Hanoi medical school classmates. The hospital's architecture was the same as Bac Lieu, but much cleaner, with glass windows, cloth mattresses, and sheets. There was a minimum of debris or dirt. After tea with Vinh's colleagues, we toured the city, including the central market where Montagnard natives sold souvenirs. These "people of the mountains" were easily distinguished from other Vietnamese by their complexions, high cheekbones, and dark robes. They carried their infants on their backs, like Native American papooses.

We saw few Americans, as the area was off-limits to U.S. personnel not on official business. How did Vinh arrange a visit to such a restricted zone? I gave a silent thanks to our friends at USAID.

Wealthy and high-ranking VN and French have used Dalat as a refreshing getaway for decades. Among those with homes in Dalat were the Diem family. Ngo Dinh Diem became prime minister in the mid–1950s. He was initially supported by the U.S., but his regime became increasingly corrupt and unable to cope with insurgents, including the Viet Cong. Diem was a bachelor. His brother's wife was Tran Le Xuan, otherwise known as Madam Nhu, who became the unofficial first lady of Vietnam. The Diem government was harsh, prompting multiple Buddhist uprisings with several self-immolations by monks, which Madam Nhu mocked as "barbecues." She remained a controversial figure. When Ngo Diem and her husband were assassinated in 1963, she went into exile.

Despite her absence from Vietnam, Madam Nhu's fiery pronouncements continued, and she was a sharp critic of American policies for decades. Vinh told us the history of the Diems as we drove through the city into the surrounding hills. Presently, we came to a deserted house nestled among several beautiful homes in the pines. At the driveway we were met by five ARVN guards. Additional soldiers were stationed in the yard and at the front door. The stucco and wood structure was a modernistic, single-story home with large bay windows, and a swimming pool and Japanese garden in the back yard.

Although of modest size, perhaps 2,500 square feet, the home was elegant. Vinh spoke to one of the guards. After a brief conversation, he unlocked the front door, ushered us inside, and accompanied us as we walked through the house. Most of the furniture had been removed, and small piles of rubbish were scattered on the varnished wood floors. We stepped past a partially unpacked crate in the master bedroom and gazed at a large painting of a handsome woman in formal attire. I immediately recognized her as the notorious Madam Nhu. None of us needed further explanations—this was the Diem home. How had Vinh gained access? The effect was eerie, as if viewing the scene of a crime. We walked through the paneled den and into the living room where stuffed leopards and the trophy head of a gaur, a large animal like a buffalo, lay on the floor, waiting to be hung over the ornate, wooden mantel. In the master bath we saw Madam Nhu's chair for makeup and hairstyling, as well as the control station of the intercom system. We exited through a sliding glass door in the bedroom to the back yard, where a tiled rectangular swimming pool was filled with brackish water and debris. A small untended Japanese garden was nearby. The yard was surrounded by pine trees and adjacent homes, which were similarly well-appointed.

Our group was silent as we explored the home. The guards were anxious for us to conclude our visit, although Vinh retained his usual calm nature, unaffected by the guards' discomfort. As we returned to the car, he gave us his thoughts of the Diems. Despite its many faults, Vinh believed their government represented order and retained much of the dignity and heritage of ancient VN and the French era. Vinh regretted the coup and the Diems' assassinations, but conceded they were probably inevitable. The regime had become increasingly repressive and corrupt. He said nothing of U.S. complicity in the killings. The remainder of our trip to the hotel was quiet, as we digested Vinh's thoughts. I was astonished he had been able to arrange the visit.

Madam Nhu (Tran Le Xuan 1924–2011) was the wife of Ngo Dinh Nhu, brother of President Ngo Dinh Diem, and de facto first lady of Vietnam. She was a nemesis to the United States during and after the war, strongly objecting to American policy. After her husband and the president were assassinated in November 1963, she lived in Europe, but railed against the U.S. until her death. But as Shakespeare wrote in *Macbeth*: "What, can the devil speak true?" Nhu cited many unpleasant truths of America's involvement in VN.

After a multicourse French dinner in the Palace's dining room, we walked to the Tulip Rouge bar for a drink but were greeted by a sign: "*NO US PERSONNEL ALLOWED*." Heeding the warning, we retired to a small bar just below the hotel for refreshments.

The evening was delightfully cool, and I opened the large windows to sample the gentle breeze that filtered through the pines. In the morning we learned we could not obtain a chopper to visit the Dalat leprosarium or Pasteur Institute, so Vinh hired a car for the day. We were propelled into the countryside by a colorful driver who sported a large mole on his left cheek from which three long hairs protruded. He was proud of his facial adornment, stroking the hairs as he drove. We motored along valleys, following train tracks, passing several fine homes like the Diem residence. Soon we were in a thick pine forest with ferns, wildflowers, and dark red soil. There were bamboo shoots and cinchona trees, some of which had been planted during Yersin's era. Between the cinchona trees nestled squat bushes bearing pods. Vinh explained the plants were the source of racin, a purgative. We ventured further into the forest, which held many tea plantations. Thousands of the plants were neatly spaced along hillsides, separated by vegetable gardens of onions, lettuce, and tomatoes, plus a trellised, creeping green squash termed "trai au hao," which all but engulfed the small huts in the fields. Many of the plantations were adorned with lovely Tudor homes. As we drove, we saw women picking tea leaves and men carrying bushels to dry. Along the road three soldiers carried a deer they had just shot.

About 35 km from Dalat is the village of Oran—the site of a dam that furnishes hydroelectric power to Saigon. A clear blue lake extends 4 km from the dam.

Returning through the conifers, we turned off the main road up a driveway to one of the tea plantations. Vinh introduced us to the owner, an elderly Chinese gentleman in white silk pajamas and black horn-rim glasses. He led us to the sorting room where a score of young girls separated the inferior lighter leaves and debris from the prized darker tea leaves, which were placed on wooden tables and collected in paper bags. Vinh bought two bags of the "noir" leaves.

Our plantation host escorted us to his home and treated us to a Chinese lunch. Bidding him adieu, we drove toward the falls, but came upon a checkpoint with a sign proclaiming: "*Warning US Personnel—You are entering an insecure area— before proceeding notify sector Hdqts. Security precautions—minimum of 2 automatic weapons and 2 grenades. Travel in daylight only.*" We were armed with cameras, but Vinh assured our safety and directed our driver to proceed down the serpentine road. After a few kilometers we came to a large gorge and the falls. Nearby was a small zoo that housed animals indigenous to Dalat—leopard, tiger, elephant, peacock, gaur, deer, wild boar, and various monkeys. From the falls, Vinh pointed out Lan Bien, the highest peak in the area.

The afternoon wore on and we returned to the Dalat airfield for our flight to Saigon. As we drove onto the strip, a Volpar Turbo Beechcraft landed and a gray-haired gentleman emerged from the plane. He was immediately surrounded by a party of dignitaries. We asked an American guard the occasion. He said, "That's Ellsworth Bunker, the new ambassador to Vietnam." The ambassador was ushered to a waiting limousine and whisked away. Luckily, we were able to hitch a ride on Bunker's plane to Saigon. Within minutes we were skimming above the Dalat hills at 180 knots. As we flew over plantations we had visited earlier, Vinh reflected, "When we return after the war, we must motor to my plantation." I didn't know if he was speaking rhetorically or indeed had property in Dalat. But his eyes held his meaning, and he quietly added that it was unlikely that he would return to the mountain retreat. Minutes passed. I asked why he worked in Bac Lieu. With his talents and reputation, I repeated what Bill Owen told me months earlier: Vinh could be medicine chief of any province, or a professor in Saigon. He smiled, "Bac Lieu is my home now. I must work for my family and my country. We have a saying: 'When the father is alive, his children's heels are red. After he dies, they are muddy.' I must make a place for my children. Otherwise, 'laissez aller'—all will be gone." He became silent and turned his head to look out the cabin window.

We arrived safely in Saigon and Vinh treated us to a Chinese dinner in Cholon, followed by a visit to a nightclub where we danced with young girls in lovely *áo dàis*. Our entertainment was cut short by the nightly 10:00 p.m. curfew.

The following morning an Air America plane flew us directly to Bac Lieu. Landing was complicated, as several gunships were parked beside the runway. A two-day divisional operation had been held, and many choppers remained at the airfield. We learned one casualty was a gunship crew chief who fell out of a chopper. His body had not been located. Thus ended our Dalat holiday: welcome back to Bac Lieu!

Chapter Sources

J. Hochgesang, T. Lawyer, and T. Stevenson. *The Psychological Effects of the Vietnam War.* 1999. https://www.eriesd.org/site/handlers/filedownload.ashx?moduleinstanceid=9526&dataid=11852&FileName=The%20Psychological%20Effects%20of%20the%20Vietnam%20War-1.pdf.

George Lepre. *Fragging: Why U.S. Soldiers Assaulted Their Officers in Vietnam.* Lubbock, TX: Texas Tech University Press, 2011.

Hamilton Gregory. "Murder in Vietnam." *Military History* 35, no. 2 (2018): 40–43.

Peter Brush. "The Hard Truth About Fragging." *Vietnam* 35, no. 2 (2018): 22–29.

R. A. Kulla, W. E. Schlenger, J. A. Fairbank, et al. *National Vietnam Veterans Readjustment Study (NVVS): Description, Current Status, and Initial PTSD Prevalence Estimates.* Triangle Park, NC: Triangle Institute, PB90–164203, 1988.

Charles R. Marmar, William Schlenger, Clare Henn-Haase, et al. "Course of Posttraumatic Stress Disorder 40 Years After the Vietnam War: Findings from the National Vietnam Veterans Longitudinal Study." *JAMA Psychiatry* 72, no. 9 (2015): 875–81.

Bruce P. Dohrenwend, J. Blake Turner, Nicholas A. Turse, et al. "Psychological Risks of Vietnam for U.S. Veterans: A Revisit With New Data and Methods." *Science* 313, no. 5789 (2006): 979–82.

———. "Continuing Controversy Over the Psychological Risk of Vietnam for U.S. Veterans." *Journal of Traumatic Stress* 20, no. 4 (2007): 449–65.

Dean G. Kilpatrick. "Confounding the Critics: The Dohrenwend and Colleagues Reexamination of the National Vietnam Veterans Readjustment Study." *Journal of Traumatic Stress* 20, no. 4 (2007): 487–83.

Richard J. McNally. "Revisiting Dohrenwend et al.'s Revisit of the National Vietnam Veterans Readjustment Study." *Journal of Traumatic Stress* 20, no. 4 (2007): 481–86.

Roger S. Mitchell. "Control of Tuberculosis." *New England Journal of Medicine* 276, no. 15 (1967): 842–8.

John F. Murray. "Mycobacterium Tuberculosis and the Cause of Consumption: From Discovery to Fact." *American Journal of Respiratory Critical Care* 169, no. 10 (2004): 1086–88.

John F. Murray, Dean E. Schraufnagel, and Philip C. Hopewell. "Treatment of Tuberculosis: A Historical Perspective." *Annals of the American Thoracic Society* 12, no. 12 (2015): 1749–59.

T. D. Brock. *Robert Koch: A Life in Medicine and Bacteriology.* Washington, D.C.: American Society for Microbiology, 1999.

John Steinbeck. "Letters From John Steinbeck." *Chicago Tribune*, February 26, 1967.

Rojelio Mejia, Jill Weatherhead, and Peter J. Hotez. "Intestinal Nematodes (Roundworms)." Chapter 286 in *Mandell, Douglas and Bennett's Principles and Practice of Infectious Diseases.* 9th ed. Edited by J. Bennett, R. Dolin, and M. J. Blaser. Philadelphia: Elsevier, 2020.

William Harris. Obituary. *Island Vegetarian: Vegetarian Society of Hawaii* 27, no. 1 (2016): 1–2.

John J. Deller, Dallas E. Smith, David T. English, et al. "Venereal Diseases." Chapter 9 in *Internal Medicine in Vietnam, Vol. II: General Medicine and Infectious Diseases.* Edited by Andre J. Ognibene and O'Neill Barrett, Jr., Washington, D.C.: U.S. Government Printing Office, 1982.

Monique Demery. *Finding the Dragon Lady: The Mystery of Vietnam's Madame Nhu.* New York: Public Affairs, 2013.

James H. Gregory. "Madame Nhu, Vietnam War Lightning Rod Dies." *New York Times*, April 26, 2011.

Shakespeare. *Macbeth.* Act 1, Scene 3.

Stanley Karnow. *Vietnam: A History.* New York: Viking Press, 1983.

12

July

Drugs, Diphtheria, and Dowling

We were elated to learn Dr. Khoung departed for military duty during our Dalat trip. Charlie promptly assumed responsibility for Ward 8 and made rounds with Linda. Many patients had not been seen for days, and no medical notes had been written for months. One elderly man was shaking with a fever and could not rise from bed. The family told us his chills had persisted for nearly a week. Charlie and Linda were disgusted with the poor care and Khoung's abandonment, but it was a welcome opportunity.

We sweated through two hot, rainless days with temperatures above 100 degrees, although clinics were busy. A female VC prisoner was brought to the ER. She was covered in mud, confused, and suffering from kidney failure, but her mental state was more complicated. She gave a story of capture and rape by ARVN soldiers, although details changed constantly, and we suspected an underlying psychosis. Her fate would be adverse as there were no facilities for dialysis or psychiatric care, especially for a prisoner.

Charlie faced another dilemma. A VC was brought by police. The man was very sick with multiple medical problems. Charlie said hospitalization was required, but the police were emphatic. "He cannot stay," an officer shouted, "He is our prisoner—he cannot stay: Give him a shot!" Charlie realized his dilemma and reluctantly ordered injection of an antibiotic. The man was promptly dragged to a waiting car. Charlie pondered the episode, knowing the patient would die, but police could claim they sought medical care.

That evening we met over drinks and discussed the attitudes of our hosts. We concluded the Vietnamese nurtured sentimental, romantic memories of the French, whereas they were wary of Americans, and our actions had not gained their respect. They maintained a kinship and fondness for the French, whom they believed understood and appreciated Vietnamese life, culture, and history. But they freely admitted the colonizers exploited their country, although the French lived with and among the people, unlike the aloof, condescending, and judgmental yanks. The Vietnamese were nostalgic of French culture, science, and medicine, whereas our modern, mechanized, and impersonal approaches were viewed with distrust. For reasons we couldn't comprehend, Vinh was unique. He evoked a different spirit, was open to new ideas, and genuinely appreciated, even wished for our help. In turn, he responded to our efforts with reciprocal generosity and friendship. We could not assess his attitudes of America's involvement in the war, but his dedication to his country and Bac Lieu was obvious. His support of our efforts was remarkable. Unfortunately, Vinh's future would be in jeopardy if his predictions were correct.

An outpost at Ba Xuyen was attacked, killing five soldiers, including the commander. The outpost was pinned down for hours until Spooky arrived. War was omnipresent and depressing, and it wasn't always clear who was winning. We focused on our delta battles, ignorant of events transpiring in the north. As we sipped our drinks, Da Nang reeled from a devastating rocket attack. The episode occurred 200 miles away, but it might have been thousands.

I accompanied Dr. Vinh, Red Cross officials, and prominent city residents for an enlightening but depressing trip to the city prison. Food, clothing, and other supplies were given to the inmates, a wretched of group 400 men and women. The civilian jail consisted of five cement structures covered by a corrugated metal roof. There were no beds or running water, and prison sentences frequently exceeded seven years. Prisoners were fed twice a day, usually rice and a fish or a meat dish. Vinh and I held sick call in a small office. Most of the patients suffered from malnutrition and parasites; several inmates had TB. There was no prison ward in the province hospital, so patients remained at the city jail without isolation facilities. A few men bore bruises and other signs of physical trauma. Vinh told me torture was commonplace, usually tightly coiling wire around arms or hands, leaving it in place for hours. We saw only bruises, and no obvious signs of torture. Each mammoth cell held up to 100 prisoners, with limited light and ventilation. Men and women peered at us like animals in cages. It was like visiting a dungeon from the past.

Other justice was equally harsh. Those convicted of capital crimes awaited the arrival of the country's sole traveling guillotine. After conviction, a province made a request to Saigon. The guillotine moved from site to site for executions, along with the executioner. I shuddered as Vinh described the grizzly process.

Among the visitors was a well-dressed matronly woman, Ba Vt Thuong, owner of the local house of prostitution. She was wealthy and owned a large section of land near the city, plus a herd of water buffalo that she rented to local farmers. A prominent member of Bac Lieu society, she donated to many charitable causes, including the jail.

Vinh introduced me to the lady, who was very gracious, although she spoke no English. She and Vinh enjoyed a laugh as Vinh asked if MILPHAP doctors could obtain a discount at her establishments. She grinned and quickly answered in the affirmative, raising two fingers to indicate the price of 200 piastres, much to the delight of those within earshot. I was spared further embarrassment as the assembled guests walked to their waiting Peugeots and Citroens. An amused Vinh smiled and patted me on the back as we departed.

The Air Force was testing a new system of night surveillance and destroy mission in the delta. A MACV officer described the deadly scenario as follows: A Martin B-57 jet equipped with infrared detectors and a sophisticated radar system flew high over canals and other routes of infiltration, followed by additional aircraft of the killer team. With its electronic equipment the B-57 could detect sampans, troop movements, and other military targets in the dark from a considerable altitude. Flying a few miles behind the B-57 was an F-100 fighter jet, carrying flares that were dropped on positions identified by the B-57. To complete the lethal trio, another ship followed with mini-cannons and rockets to attack targets lit by the flares. Thus, a sampan carrying VC was sighted by a plane high overhead without lights or sound, arousing no attention. Within a minute or two, the enemy was under the glare of flares dropped by the second ship. Before they could flee, they were fired upon by the third aircraft. It was an awesome system of sophisticated detection and killing.

We received a new team member, Spc. Davis, a burly, friendly fellow, who perspired heavily as a new in-country arrival. He had a much-needed talent—lab technician. Within a few days he befriended the VN technician, who was happy to have him perform most of the laboratory studies, an echo of Vinh's earlier observations.

I held another sad, frustrating clinic. One of the hospital workers brought her five-year-old to the adult clinic. When I saw the child carried into the exam room, I was irritated. The employee should know not to bring a child to the adult unit. But as the nearly lifeless child was placed on the table, I knew she was moribund. Before I could perform even a cursory exam, she died. Between sobs and wails, the mother clutched the dead child to her breast. The girl had been ill with fever, sleepiness, and "stiff neck" for several days. But only today the mother believed she should come to the hospital. A tragic story, and I was embarrassed. It took several minutes to clear the room of the grieving mother to resume clinic.

I was roused at 4:00 a.m. The gate guard apologetically said, "Sir, there's a call for you." "But I'm not on call tonight," I answered. The guard responded, "Yes, but Dr. Tot said, 'Call Dr. Carlson—patient wounded—I can't fix.'"

The patient was a boy who had been wounded by a 105 mm shell. There were large entrance and exit wounds of the back. As we finished surgery, Vinh and I went directly to the airport for a meeting of province medicine chiefs in Can Tho. We were greeted by John Marsh, who issued a strange greeting: "Welcome; Great day—stick around for the fireworks."

Vinh introduced me to other medicine chiefs, head nurses, and midwives. I noted I was the only MILPHAP physician in attendance. A Saigon delegation represented the MOH, including several regional directors, among them Dr. Chung, a talkative fellow in a wrinkled pinstripe suit, smoking a cigar. Chung said he was responsible for public health in the delta.

The first three rows of the room were equipped with headsets for translation. After the national anthem was played over a scratchy loudspeaker, Dr. Khoa, the Region IV senior health officer, conducted the meeting. Dr. Chung was seated next to him. The morning sessions dealt with hospital supply, although no one addressed the loss of equipment from Saigon.

Politics quickly crept into the agenda. A vote was held on whether a midwife could be appointed province medicine chief. The province chiefs, all doctors, voted no. The midwives and nurses voted yes. The measure was defeated. Male dominance flourished.

The morning session adjourned, and we walked to a Chinese restaurant. I was seated across from Doug, Marsh and Dr. Chung, who proceeded to consume two

Scotch and waters. As I struggled with chopsticks, Dr. Chung asked innocently, "I understand you have a contraceptive, so-called loop clinic in Bac Lieu." I glanced across the table at Doug, who raised his eyebrows but didn't say anything.

"We see a few patients," I replied, as noncommittal as possible. I tried to avoid a scene, especially in the presence of MOH representatives. As the sailor refrain goes: Don't make waves among larger craft—their wake may swamp you.

But Chung persisted, "You know such things are against Vietnamese law. In fact, birth control and population problems have been discussed by the ministry. As far as I know, there is no change in the law."

Uh-oh, I thought, as I meekly replied, "I'm distressed to hear that, as many patients ask for help." I tried to obtain some cover, adding, "I believe Dr. Guttmacher was recently in Vietnam and spoke with the ministry on this topic."

Dr. Alan F. Guttmacher (1898–1974), a prominent obstetrician, was president of Planned Parenthood (PP) for many years. PP was the culmination of work by Margaret Sanger (1879–1966), a social activist and nurse pioneer in the U.S. birth control movement, although she embraced theories of eugenics. Guttmacher travelled to VN in the 1960s, promoting the concept of family planning. I thought his name might defuse the situation.

Dr. Chung responded, "I don't see Vietnam has any population problem which need concern us. Our land can support a large population. And we are of French heritage, which prohibits such practice. Surely Doctor, you don't think birth control is needed here?" he asked with certainty as he finished his third Scotch.

By now Doug was giving me the high sign to "cool it," so I responded with the tact I could muster, but passion ultimately ruled. "Most women have several children and come with husbands to limit their families. Contraception isn't the answer to all the country's health problems but should be available if requested. A woman who…" I stopped, as I realized I had already said too much.

Doug started to speak but was interrupted by Dr. Chung. "Ah, but you don't consider the future. We need many children for soldiers to fight. Family planning, as you call it, sounds noble and good, but won't work here. We Orientals like big families—it is our tradition. Besides, if we improve people's health, more infants will be saved, and we will have a bigger, stronger nation."

With that comment, lunch concluded and Doug and I were relieved the discussion had not become uglier. We returned to the lecture hall for the afternoon's program. The discussion turned to midwives and the three-year curriculum of midwife training. Each province had its own educational program. Newly minted midwives, reluctant to remain in the hamlets, migrated to Can Tho or Saigon, where they established lucrative private practices. The discussion was heated, but the officials conceded they were unable to control the distribution of midwives.

The next agenda item was the BCG vaccination program. MOH decreed all newborns should receive BCG. But for the 8,000 infants born yearly in the delta, less than 10 percent received the vaccine. The problem was logistical. The vaccine must be refrigerated, and most rural areas lacked electrical power, so children not born in province hospitals or larger regional facilities were not vaccinated. Attendees had no solution to the problem.

The BCG vaccine was developed after World War I by Calmette and Guerin, contemporaries of Yersin at the Pasteur Institute in Paris. Given to newborns, the vaccine provides good protection for severe forms of TB such as meningitis, although it is less effective to prevent pulmonary TB, the most common manifestation. BCG is still utilized in countries in which TB is endemic. Recently, the vaccine has been studied as an immune modulator in the management of COVID-19.

In the final session, John Marsh discussed the impact of MILPHAP teams on provincial health in a farewell address, as he was returning to civilian life. Even the restrained province medicine chiefs gave John a robust round of applause as the meeting adjourned.

USAID benefited by several dedicated individuals, such as Drs. Moncrief, Douglas, and Marsh. Unfortunately, they were hampered by bureaucracy, governmental corruption, graft, and especially the war.

Two children with diphtheria had been admitted in my absence. We attempted to trace contacts and obtain throat cultures. The kids were very sick. One girl had the "bull neck" and facial paralysis described in textbooks, and both exhibited the classic dirty-gray membrane in the throat and unpleasant fetor. These were the first cases of diphtheria I'd seen, as immunization had wiped out the disease in the States. Diphtheria is highly contagious and carries a significant risk of death, often due to the bacterium's toxin. My father's younger sister died of diphtheria in the early 1900s of cardiac complications.

Diphtheria is infection by *Corynebacterium diphtheriae*. Diphtheria, also termed "throat distemper," has been known for thousands of years, and "Egyptian throat ulcers" were described by Hippocrates. In the 18th and early 19th centuries, American colonies and Europe experienced many outbreaks. Pierre Bretonneau, a giant of French medicine, coined the term "diphtheria" from the Greek word for skin or hide, referring to the thick membrane that develops in the posterior pharynx. Bretonneau was ahead of his time, believing diphtheria and other infectious diseases were transmitted by "morbid seeds," although the germ theory of infections was decades in the future when Frederich Loeffler and Robert Koch identified the microbes of diphtheria, TB, and cholera. Treatment of diphtheria was primitive, with death usually from respiratory failure. The disease is especially virulent in children, with tragic endings. A child may appear to improve, only to die suddenly of a cardiac arrhythmia. Diphtheria, like tetanus, produces a powerful toxin that affects several organs, including the heart. Antitoxin therapy has been available since the 1890s.

Widespread immunization essentially eradicated diphtheria in many countries, using DPT (diphtheria, whooping cough or pertussis, and tetanus) vaccine. Many cases were reported in VN during the 1960s, none in U.S. troops. The two girls ultimately survived with antibiotics and close nursing care.

Agricultural as well as medical assistance were provided by USAID. Over lunch Pete Peterson, the affable USAID agricultural advisor, gave me an update on delta rice production. The province yielded more than 200,000 annual tons of rice, although 30 percent was lost in milling. As I learned earlier, the yield was far less than in the United States, but rice was very important for civilian and military use, and a dietary staple. Each ARVN soldier was issued one-half kilo per day. Before the war, VN produced more rice than it utilized, exporting excess to other countries. In 1967 there was no surplus, due to substantial losses to the VC, a major pillar of their war effort. I'd soon learn the VC's tenacity to maintain canal blocks to confiscate rice and other products.

I documented my VN sojourn with a journal and 16 mm film. Some of the footage I shot was utilized for a movie I made with the AMA to promote the VPVN program. I also played cinematographer for Jack Redman. When he discovered I had a camera, he had film shipped from New Mexico. I'd photograph him operating, treating patients, and interacting with MACV officers. The exposed film was returned to New Mexico where it was shown on local TV. I didn't know the reason for the promotional effort, until Jack told he had run for Congress and was considering another try.

Jack Redman, MD, was a prominent physician in Albuquerque, New Mexico. A family physician, he graduated from the University of Colorado School of Medicine, served in the Navy, and unsuccessfully ran for Congress in 1962 and 1964. He was a popular local figure and had a long association with the University of New Mexico (Jack C. Redman, MD, 1924–1994).

Dr. Alan Homay departed on the morning 'bou. During his tenure in Bac Lieu, he participated in a variety of medical tasks—pediatric and medicine clinics, ER duties, assistant surgeon, and on-call. He was popular with the VN staff and worked

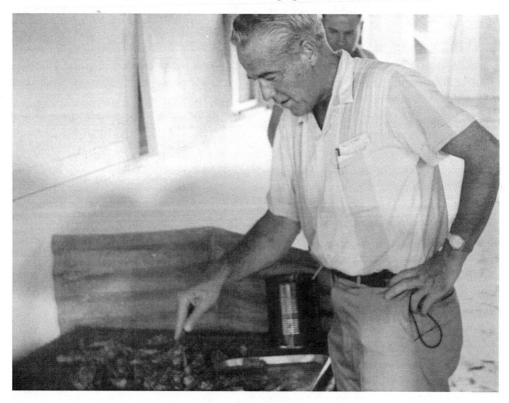

Dr. Jack Redman at MACV BBQ.

quietly and humbly. Alan Homay (originally Ali Homoyounpour) was born in Teheran. He immigrated to Europe and lived in Switzerland before the Rotary Club of California sponsored his move to the United States in 1951. He practiced in California and Arizona before retiring. He died in Sun City, Arizona (A. Homay, MD, 1919–1995).

One evening Vinh asked if we would like to go downtown for "something special." Jim had inquired if opium smoking remained popular in VN. Vinh told Jim the practice was widespread, particularly among Chinese, and promised a visit to an opium parlor.

That rainy night we were driven by Vinh to a home near the police chief's house where we were invited inside and escorted to a white plastered room, which held a pendulum clock and a dove in a small wicker cage in one corner. Presently, an elderly gentleman with a long, white beard and silk pajamas greeted us and exchanged words with Vinh. Our host asked us to follow him. After a short hallway we entered a chamber approximately 12 feet square, lit by a solitary flickering kerosene lamp. The center of the room was occupied by a large, low cherry table bearing the lamp. A middle-aged man reclined on the table, assembling two pipes, each about 18 inches in length. On one pipe a small metal bowl was positioned midway. Several metal probes and a glass of water were placed near the lamp. We were told the cherry table is called an Oriental bed. It was large enough for three or four individuals to recline simultaneously. In one corner of the room was a pile of rice hull bags, atop which two children sat, watching intently. There was a single boarded window. We could hear the rain outside.

I describe our narcotic adventure in the first person, avoiding uncomfortable or embarrassing remarks of my colleagues.

The man on the table invited me to remove my shoes and lie next to him, parallel but separated by the lamp. Vinh said the pipe paraphernalia are termed "Mam Den," and that I would shortly be "introduced" to "Ong Hut," literally, Mr. Pipe. The man on the table began a complex process of preparing Mr. Pipe for action and told me to following his instructions. My comrades snapped pictures and watched with a combination of anxiety and curiosity.

"Hut a phiem," or opium smoking, has been part of Asian life for centuries. Although illegal, it remained a fixture of the culture and was tolerated in many countries. My thoughts turned to the nearby police chief's house. At that time Laos had the most permissive legislation regarding opium, and Vinh said the evening's supply of opium was smuggled into VN by airplane from Laos. The crudely refined drug is a dark, syrupy substance held in small glass vials. The man opened a vial and teased out a glob approximately one-half inch in diameter, using one of the metal probes, twirling the material like cotton candy. He heated the mass over the lamp until it became a light golden color, bubbling slightly, then quickly stuffed the opium into the small, deep bowl of the pipe. There were two pipes, but only one bowl, which was attached to the pipe with wetted strips of cloth. The first pipe was an elaborately carved hardwood cylinder with Chinese characters, decorated with brass fittings around the bowl's seat. At the end of the pipe was the mouthpiece, also made of wood. The other pipe was less fancy—a piece of clear plastic tubing, stained brown

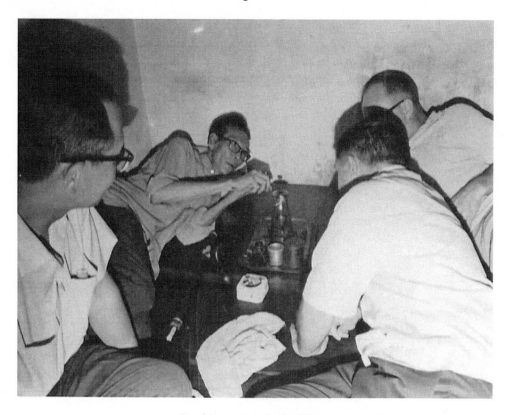

Smoking opium in Bac Lieu.

by prolonged use. The tube was connected to a standard pipe mouthpiece. At intervals throughout the evening the bowl was transferred from one pipe to the other.

Once the opium is placed in the bowl, the pipe is inverted and held over the lamp. Small curetting motions of the probe tease the opium into the proper shape, as the bowl is held above the flame to retain the viscosity of the opium. The subject deeply inhales the dark smoke which arises during this process. The acrid odor was strong and permeated the room.

The instructor told me to breathe deeply ("aspiration fortament"). Two or three puffs are taken, and the inspired air is retained as long as possible to allow exchange of the smoke in the lungs. Pictures were snapped as I sampled the fruit of the poppy. After a few puffs, I lay back on the table with closed eyes. I noted no effects but was relaxed.

I felt nothing after the first pipe. But after two or three pipes I was "changed," and after the fourth pipe I was "floating; serene and happy."

Nearly an hour passed and I was in my own world. I felt unwell, but was able to interact with my surroundings. I recalled Vinh said a vial of opium cost approximately 500 piastres, and users typically consume 800–1,000 piastres of opium a day. To conserve the precious opium, the bowl is scraped clean after use, and the contents saved. The cloth strips that held the bowl to the pipe are soaked in water and the fluid drunk, producing a cheap but less potent effect of the drug. During the night's adventure less than one vial of opium was consumed.

Over time I became more lucid. Dr. Vinh explained in earlier times wealthy opium users had servants throw pebbles on the roof, producing a sound similar to that of rain, as gentle stimuli are pleasing to the narcotized. No stones were needed, as there was a steady downpour outside.

Vinh ultimately prodded us to leave and I stumbled out of the house into his vehicle, forgetting to pay my respects to the host. The ride to the compound's back gate was short, and soon we were in the officers' club where the evening's movie was concluding. I staggered to the bar. The movie featured the Foreign Legion, but the action appeared to be in slow motion—the natives' attack seemed interminable, and a lance's flight required several seconds. I remained for a few minutes, but a heavy fatigue overtook me, and I retreated to my hooch.

Although I was tired, rest did not come easily. Each time I closed my eyes the last scene of the movie was before me. If I tightly shut my eyes, I saw a kaleidoscope of multiple colors. I experienced waves of nausea and vertigo, but sleep ultimately came.

The next morning, I attended clinic but was "hung over" most of the day. Fortunately, the hospital and clinics were quiet. At the officers' club that evening we concluded our brief acquaintance with "Ong Hut" was a unique experience but none of us planned a future sampling of "tears of the poppy."

Opium is a product of the seed capsule of the poppy *Papaver somniferum*. The raw, syrupy extract is a powerful drug and can easily be refined to morphine and heroin. Opium poppies have been cultivated since at least 1580 BCE. Egyptians named the product "juice of the poppy" and there were huge poppy fields near Thebes. Greeks and Romans cultivated the plant, and it is speculated Alexander the Great's soldiers distributed poppy seeds to much of the known world. By the 7th century, Arab traders brought opium to India and China. However, large-scale opium abuse in China did not develop until much later, fostered by the Portuguese and later the British. Imports of opium to China by the British East India Company were hugely profitable, and England fought and won two wars to continue the Chinese trade. The practice continued into the 20th century.

When the communists assumed control of China in the 1940s, Mao's regime instituted a vigorous program to eliminate opium abuse. Dealers and importers were arrested, and hundreds were executed; drug users received mandatory sentences. Drug abuse in China was markedly reduced and the opium trade moved south to the Golden Triangle of Laos, Thailand, and Myanmar. As Vinh noted, the opium we smoked was smuggled into VN through Laos. American troops discovered opium and many soldiers became heroin addicts as well as abused other drugs. In America the common term for opium is "dope," derived from the Old English "dyppan," or Dutch "doop," for sauce.

In addition to the deluge of war and medical crises, weather frequently dominated our lives. Heat alternated with the monsoon. In July, air hung heavily over the city with soaring humidity and temperatures. By the afternoon the sky could no longer contain its burden, and a furious wind coupled with rain struck, drenching us for several hours. Patients fled as the monsoon hit. The compound frequently lost power and soldiers on duty were forced to use flashlights, creating an eerie glow from the guard posts. Humidity affected everything and clothes rotted. Our hot boxes were lifesavers to protect valuables.

Don Robinson prepared to leave Bac Lieu for the last time and become a civilian. He would return to Pennsylvania to resume teaching or pursue hospital administration. Don's efforts were invaluable. His skill and enthusiasm kept the team functioning, as he managed a budget of $400,000, directed building programs, and was the senior officer for the enlisted corpsmen. Vinh held a dinner party in his honor and the next morning we loaded Don and his baggage on the 'bou for Saigon.

During the year, I received briefings on multiple medical and military issues. I also received medical bulletins, many of which were of little interest to me. However, in a batch of military mail, I read a paper by an Army psychiatrist, which profoundly altered my views, and was a groundbreaking study. The manuscript was "Psychological Aspects of the Year in Vietnam," by Dr. Jerome Dowling. He identified three phases of a soldier's emotional response to VN: a period of apprehensive enthusiasm; followed by resignation; and finally, an interval of anxious apprehension. During the first weeks, a soldier is energetic and excited by his new environment. This emotion quickly gives way to disillusionment as he observes the dirt and poverty of the country, and the reality of military duties. Death is suddenly a very real possibility. Dowling wrote, "In one particular battalion a newly assigned PFC has a 50–50 chance of surviving the year based on the battalion's first year statistics. These facts lead to anxiety. Others react differently, and some commanders become obsessed with duty and demand strict obedience." Dowling cited one officer who required his staff to salute his helicopter, reminding me of the colonel's edicts to wash Jeeps daily.

He continued, "Enthusiasm gives way to anxiety but also resignation and depression. A ten-to-fifteen-pound weight loss is common within the first few months of deployment. Sleep is affected by daily danger, anxiety and nightly artillery fire, the weather or other factors." I nodded agreement, as his narrative continued:

> Social interaction is limited … activities such as volley ball, cards, cameras, tape recording, reading … are utilized in fits and starts as depression waxes and wanes…. Officers and NCOs … show more than the usual depressive symptomatology, marked by sleeplessness, anorexia, exaggerated states of fear, and, in many cases, an attempt to compensate with increased alcohol intake. These men are not sick enough to warrant psychiatric evacuation, nor do they respond miraculously to a 2–3-day hospitalization. Usually a complex administrative-medical dialogue ensues with varying outcomes—the most common being a down-grading of job responsibility. Most of us spend these months doing our job, looking forward to making arrangements for R&R, leave, or TDY [temporary duty]. The R&R and leave have their own prodromal euphoria and anxiety prior to departure. On return there is a subsequent week to ten-day depression…. Lastly, as DEROS [date of expected return from overseas] approaches, there is another interval of anxious apprehension…. Suicide is also a risk.

I was astounded how Dowling's comments coincided not only with my personal reactions, but observations of others. The report gave me insight and allayed some of my apprehensions. Knowledge is a potent weapon against fear. But for many soldiers the emotion was palpable. Men were being injured and killed faster than they were replaced. I wondered if Secretary McNamara and President Johnson's promise of a "significant" increase in troop strength would offset these realities. I was safer in the delta, but there was no hiding from fate. The omnipresence of war seared psychological scars upon all.

Dowling's article paved the way for identification of PTSD and presaged the Veterans Readjustment Study. In his book "*US Army Psychiatry in Vietnam*," Dr. Norman Camp cited Dowling as "one of the first psychiatrists to describe the psycho-social stressors that commonly affected troops serving in a combat division, as well as patterns of maladjustment and dysfunction." The concept of fear, leading to anxiety and ultimately PTSD, was emerging. When I read Dowling's paper in 1967, I could not appreciate how prescient his comments were to become.

The colonel's behavior could have been culled from Dowling's descriptions. The latest edict stated anyone without a mess card would not be served in the mess hall; and no Bermuda shorts, shower shoes, or baseball caps would be tolerated on the compound.

A four-day divisional operation was held, which became a four-day flop. Intelligence predicted VC in large numbers, but four days searching rice paddies, blowing up hamlets, and air strikes yielded 10 VC at a cost of two million dollars, proving war is an inefficient endeavor, especially with poor intelligence.

Although ARVN activities were frequently unsuccessful, the VC could attack or impose terror at will. Two health workers in Gia Rai were assassinated, followed by the prompt resignations of the remainder of the staff. Recruitment for the clinic had taken Vinh several months.

Rain continued with a predictable pattern: heat and humidity increased until afternoon, when wind and rain would persist for several hours.

Despite weather, casualties continued: One man was shot through the face. Another stepped on a mine, amputating his left leg. Charlie and Vinh operated on a third victim, a head wound with uncontrollable bleeding, which was ultimately fatal. The torrent of injured matched the rain.

Army news reported 283 U.S. soldiers died the prior week, with more than 1,100 wounded. ARVN losses were listed as 144 killed and 383 wounded. These were horrendous numbers, but it didn't seem equitable our losses should be greater than VN soldiers. I thought, "This is no longer a war fought by Vietnamese." The United States was hobbled by an increasingly reluctant ally. The pattern continued throughout the late 1960s and early 1970s, with further erosion of American support. The VC were playing a waiting game: as Saigon dallied, U.S. soldiers died.

Dr. Stark left for Da Nang to visit his son Tom in a combat location, as Steve prepared to fly to Hong Kong for R&R. I would visit the British Crown Colony in August.

I admitted a Cambodian boy with massive gastrointestinal bleeding, likely from typhoid. We pleaded with the family to donate blood. They refused. Ultimately, Jim and I each gave a unit. There was something mystical about blood; it was prized. A unit from a "professional donor" in a downtown center cost 5,000 piastres, about $45, representing several months' wages. We never learned why the family refused. The boy died despite massive intravenous fluids, and our two units.

Doctor Vinh presented certificates of the Red Cross first aid course to high school seniors. Jim Parker and Mariana taught the course. Among the graduates was a handsome lad I had seen in clinic with symptoms of a common cold. When I examined his chest, there were numerous cup marks and acupunctures by a local Chinese practitioner. The boy was among the top of his class. Unfortunately, the training did not discuss the ineffectiveness of spiritualism. At least his clean, white shirt hid the cup marks. Vinh was very scornful of folk practices, although beliefs died slowly. Cupping as well as pinching, lacerations, and other measures were very common in Vietnam, employed for virtually any malady. Heated metal or glass cylinders closed at one end were applied to the skin. The typical results were small bruises or ecchymoses due to distortion of the skin and capillary damage. Although the scientific merits are unproven, cupping is still available throughout the world—including the United States. To our amazement, many of the hospital employees' kids bore cup marks.

The evening's movie was terrible, and we assembled in Capt. Everett Covington's hooch for his irreverent commentary on American and ARVN wartime actions. The skits were funny, like Tom Needham's "doctors' therapy sessions," but exposed unpleasant truths of behavior and attitudes.

Tonight's colorful dialogue featured the fearless ARVN cavalry and intrepid American advisors chasing VC desperados. In one scene a few VC bandits shoot at ARVN and U.S. troops from a tree line. The advisor, "Burt Lambaster," calls in air support and a fleet of choppers lays waste to the area, including a small hut owned by farmer, "Nguyen van Poor." The hut is destroyed, and Nguyen's mother is shot, along with several chickens and hogs. As the smoke clears, an ARVN officer asks Nguyen the whereabouts of the VC. The dumbfounded farmer pleads ignorance, to which the

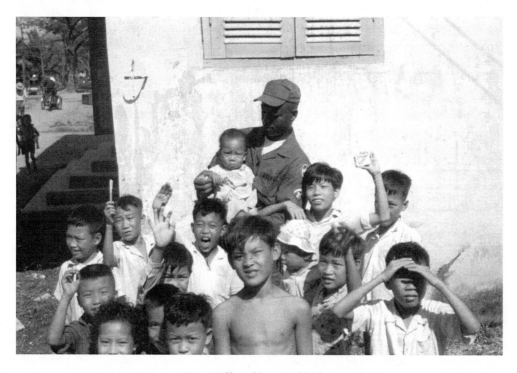

Spc. Hill and hospital kids.

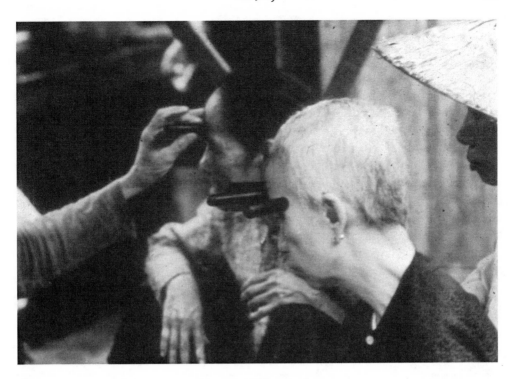

Cupping folk remedy.

officer questions how many VC were involved. The farmer replies, "Two or three." Meanwhile, ARVN troops ransack what remains of the hut, confiscating bananas and bags of rice. The officer continues his query: "Surely there were more—perhaps a platoon?" The simple farmer has no idea what constitutes a platoon, and replies, "Yes, I guess." Lambaster approaches and the farmer asks him, "What about my house, my hogs, my injured mother?" The farmer continues his plea, "What can you do?"

The American replies, "That's the trouble with you damn people—don't you realize what we're doing? We're making the land safe and helping folks like you. Aren't you grateful?"

Soon the ARVN troops and the advisors depart in their APCs, tossing Coke bottles and cigarette butts onto the road as the bewildered farmer places his bleeding mother on a cart drawn by a water buffalo. He arrives at the province hospital, where the confused farmer is greeted by a uniformed American doctor.

That evening the farmer returns to find two VC in the remains of his hut. "Hello, old friend," says one of the fighters. "I see the bloodthirsty Americans destroyed your home. We came to help as soon as possible and will rebuild your house. We'll get those imperialistic scoundrels. In the meantime, can we store our recoilless rifle ammunition in your hut?"

Cov related his tale with embellishments and Western dialect. His story was humorous, but tragic, illustrating the strained relationships between locals, ARVN, and American advisors. The VC had a tremendous propaganda machine—living with and aiding the people. But they taxed, exacted tributes, and conscripted people into service. So-called friendly ARVN forces accompanied by U.S. firepower destroyed property and injured or killed civilians. Restitution sometimes occurred but was slow and incomplete. The Americans were the aloof force behind the destruction with no sympathy or rapport with the locals. ARVN soldiers looted and confiscated property. Winning the "hearts and minds" was a difficult, if not impossible, task. In Cov's story, there were no heroes, and the peasant suffered from all combatants. The narrative was an accurate but sad parable.

Winning a guerrilla war without local support is impossible—I now suspected sooner or later the VC would be successful.

There was always a new tragedy—this time it was drowning. A man and his son were found in a canal. Their lifeless bodies were brought by the family, who cradled the faces and tearfully spoke to them. But both were dead. It took several minutes to clear the ER of the wailing family. Vinh poked his head in the door and asked if the two had been thrown in the water with hands tied behind their backs, a common practice of the VC. We never learned how they drowned.

Spooky was overhead later that night, as a local outpost had been attacked. We received four casualties and Drs. Redman and Vinh spent the following day in surgery. Jim had a frustrating night on call as he treated three patients who attempted suicide. Unfortunately, restocking emergency items was usually incomplete and haphazard. Jim feverishly opened packs of supplies, only to discover they lacked vital components, a commonplace situation. The problem was not isolated to the ER, or at night. The developer solution for X-rays had not been reordered for weeks and films were useless. The refrigerator that houses vaccines and penicillin had run out of gas—spoiling several boxes of precious medications. I thought of Vinh's comments of workers' lack of responsibility. I could never comprehend such behavior, another Bac Lieu enigma.

Jim treated two "phong" (burn) patients, only to be followed by two more. The first set were related to a gasoline spill from an outboard motor. The mother and young boy were critically burned, and both died. The other patients were victims of a cookstove explosion. Fortunately, their injuries were less severe. Injuries of war competed with civilian trauma.

Vinh and I visited a hamlet to review a new maternity-dispensary. Returning in his Land Rover, we passed rice paddies. Water buffalo and farmers trod through watery fields and peasants waved as we passed. Vinh asked if I knew how rice was planted and harvested. I replied my knowledge was rudimentary. He stopped the car and we walked to a mud and palm-frond hut that bordered a small paddy. The paddy was filled with green shoots about three-feet high. A bronzed man with powerful trunk and biceps was pulling up the shoots in bunches, tying them together and tossing them onto the bank.

Vinh pointed to the farmer and said, "See how he collects packets of shoots and carefully wraps them." He continued, "In May or June the rice grains are scattered over the paddies near the farmer's home where they can be nurtured. In a month or so the sprouts will have grown to the height you see them here. These are the stock that will be used to plant the large paddies. By now the rains have partially filled the paddies and the workers take the packets of sprouts and plant them. Each bunch is inserted in the mud by hand, about a foot apart."

In the distance I could see whole families standing in knee-deep water, bending to plant each cluster into the soggy earth, packing the mud with their feet. It was backbreaking, tedious work.

"This is called 'cay lun'," added Vinh. "The original sowing of the grains in the paddies is termed 'tam ma.' It is a way of life for these people; they have been doing it for centuries. The rice requires five or six months to mature. At the time of the new year it is harvested, also by hand. Then it is threshed, milled, and taken to cities to be sold. The husks are used for animal food and fuel."

We waved at the farmers, climbed into the car, and continued down the road. Vinh was quiet. After a kilometer or so, he turned onto a narrow lane bordered by palm trees. The lane ended at an enclosure surrounded by an ornate, rusting fence that held a cement shrine. We left the car, Vinh opened the gate, and we stood in front of two cement and white marble tombs. They were separated by an edifice of tile and crumbling stone steps. Atop one catafalque was chiseled: Tran Trinh Trach, 1872–1942.

Except for the marble and tile, the area was unkempt, with shrubs, weeds, and debris scattered among broken pieces of cement and tile. Resting on one of the tombs was a cracked ceramic pot that once held flowers.

The solitude of the scene was suddenly interrupted by two jet fighters that screamed overhead less than 150 feet above us. I could clearly see the faces of the pilots, as well as the rockets and bombs strapped beneath the wings. Once again, it was quiet.

After a moment, Vinh remarked, "In the olden times Ong [Mr.] Trach was a wealthy man who helped the people of Bac Lieu. He owned much land. But as one so

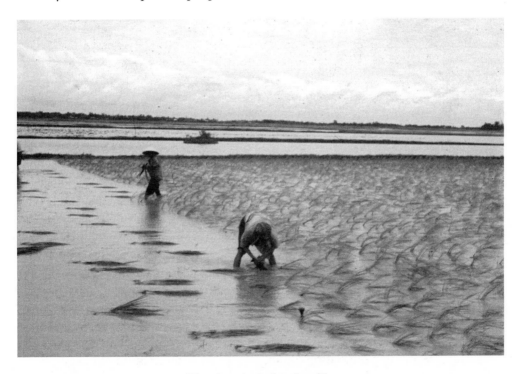

Planting rice in local paddy.

powerful, he was hated by many. In Vietnam we say respectfully of such brave men: 'Trau gia khong so dao phai'—the old buffalo is not afraid of the knife."

I asked Vinh if he ever met Ong Trach. "Yes, yes—I was his doctor and treated both he and his wife. You see her there—she died of cholera in 1947." He pointed to the marble tomb on the left.

"And what became of his family and their land?" I asked.

"He had many sons, although none as powerful as their venerable father. He was very wise—you know, in the Orient the eldest son must build a suitable tomb for his father.... It was done—but..." Vinh sighed, "See it now, 'laissez-faire'." He looked sadly around the shrine, with the crumbling cement stained by vegetation, the rusty fence and iron gate, and vines encircling the designs on the tombs.

He walked to the tomb of Ong Trach and sat on a corner. "After the time of the French, the Vietnamese government took away most of the land of the Trach descendants. The portions have been divided and redivided many times." He made a clicking sound with his tongue and shook his head, "The legacy is no more."

We returned to his car and continued our journey. He remained pensive, but said his parents were also landowners. Doubtless, they suffered the series of land reforms which destroyed the heritage of the landed gentry in Vietnam such as the Trach family. Vinh was clearly moved by thoughts of their fate. The remainder of our trip was silent. He dropped me at the compound's gate and drove off without further comment.

Dr. Stark returned from Cam Ran Bay after spending the weekend with his marine son, who had been wounded a few days earlier. The soldier was in his tent cleaning his weapon. His buddy opened the tent flap as a sniper fired. The bullet grazed his cheek—an inch difference could have been fatal.

The great intestinal epidemic of Bac Lieu infected the compound. A dozen GIs were sick with fever, vomiting, and diarrhea. Although ill, the soldiers were not critical, and no one was evacuated. After some investigation, we discovered the source—the ice cream machine in the EM club. Ice milk and water were premixed and added to the device. A sergeant discovered the Vietnamese mess personnel were using water from a tap near the NCO latrine, a non-potable source. The GIs improved within two days.

There was heavy drinking in the officers' club, and several officers stumbled to their hooches "in their cups." By 11:00 p.m. the room was nearly deserted. I was relaxed and typed my daily entries, alone, except for a gray, medium-sized rat with a depigmented tail. The animal ventured from a recess behind the piano. After satisfying himself I meant no harm, he ran to the bar, which was littered with potato chips and popcorn. The Paddy Rat Lounge was aptly named.

Jim departed for Saigon to learn more of the loop clinic's fate. Vinh drove Charlie and me to a district health station. During the trip I furthered my education on rice farming as we stopped at Lang Trong to see a rice mill. The owner, Ong King, proudly showed us his facility. We saw belt-driven shakers and separators powered by diesel engines, all in very serviceable condition. He happily demonstrated separation of rice and its preparation for shipment to Saigon in burlap bags. Workers scurried about, respectfully discharging the owner's orders. We were treated to an impromptu meal of catfish, shrimp, crab, and a variety of vegetables, as well as the ever-present cognac.

I spent another eventful evening in the ER, treating a woman who had ingested an unknown substance. She was lying on the exam table as I arrived, immobile, with shallow breathing interrupted by coughing and vomiting. Her mother wailed loudly as she dabbed Chinese medicine on the patient's chest and back. No one had tried to clear the airway of secretions, start an IV, or check the woman's blood pressure, which was dangerously low. She was in coma and had no response to pain. My exam of her lungs confirmed she had aspirated, with bilateral pneumonia. I started an IV, administered antibiotics, and inserted an oral airway. Her chances were poor, even in an American intensive care unit. But I was appalled with the lack of care prior to my arrival, and cursed the ER staff under my breath, recalling Vinh's comments on duty and responsibility.

As I finished, a cyclo arrived bearing a man with multiple wounds. He was a mass of injuries and covered in mud. I initially thought he was dead until I examined him. His eyes suddenly opened and looked at me with malevolence. One glance and I knew he was not happy to be treated by the American Bac Si. He came from VC territory via sampan and cyclo. I called to start the generator and summon Dr. Vinh.

A few minutes later, Vinh shuffled in, a cigarette dangling from his lips, his rain-soaked shirt partially unbuttoned. As usual, he showed little emotion but worked quickly to evaluate the wounds. Surgery was delayed, as the key to the operating suite couldn't be found, forcing us to stand in the rain alongside the patient on a litter. Ultimately, surgery commenced, and required three hours. During the final half-hour, the generator failed, and we were in darkness except for flashlights. Vinh didn't complain but operated silently in the feeble light. As he closed the abdomen, he remarked, "Tonight we operate like VC doctors." The operating room was still. The only sound was the anesthetist's gas machine. Vinh completed suturing the skin, removed his gown, and walked into the rainy darkness to his car.

Chapter Sources

Robert A. Dovie and David N. Tobey. "Clinical Features of Diphtheria in the Respiratory Tract." *JAMA* 242, no. 20 (1979): 2197–201.

Peter C. English. "Diphtheria and Theories of Infectious Disease: Centennial Appreciation of the Critical Role of Diphtheria in the History of Medicine." *Pediatrics* 76, no. 1 (1985): 1–9.

R. H. Semple, trans. *Memories of Diphtheria: From the Writings of Bretonneau, Guersant, Trousseau, Bouchut, Empis, and Daviot.* London: New Sydenham Society, 1859.

Jack Curry Redman. Oral History Collection, 1947–1994. New Mexico Health Historical Collection, UNM Health Sciences Library and Informatics Center.

Joseph D. Sapira. "Speculations Concerning Opium Abuse and World History." *Perspectives in Biology and Medicine* 18, no. 3 (1975): 379–96.

Hans Derks. "Opium Production and Consumption in China." In *History of the Opium Problem: The Assault of the East, ca. 1600–1950* (pp. 643–708). Leiden: Brill, 2012.

R. K. Newman. "Opium Smoking in Late Imperial China: A Reconsideration." *Modern Asian Studies* 29, no. 4 (1994): 765–94.

Jerome J. Dowling. "Psychologic Aspects of the Year in Vietnam." *US Army Vietnam Medical Bulletin* 40, no. 3 (1967): 45–48.

Diagnostic and Statistical Manual of Mental Disorders: DSM-III-R. Washington, D.C.: American Psychiatric Association, 1987.

N. Camp. *U.S. Army Psychiatry in the Vietnam War: New Challenges in Extended Counterinsurgency Warfare.* Washington, D.C.: Bordon Institute, 2015.

13

August

Daily Triumphs and Failures

Rain created huge puddles in the paths to the hospital. Hospital staff enjoyed watching the cyclos and motorcycles traverse the larger puddles, often with amusing results.

A battalion-sized group of North VN troops was sighted near the Ba Xuyen border. If true, it would be the first presence of North VN regulars this far south. There was a similar report earlier, but it was merely a VC cadre. Meanwhile, the VC shelled the Soc Trang airfield with 75 mm recoilless weapons, and two ARVN outposts, Vi Tranch and Ca Mao, were attacked: Further escalation of delta fighting.

Jim returned from Saigon, and Steve from his Hong Kong R&R. Both had interesting tales of their journeys. While in Saigon, Jim met a physician who had been assigned to a MILPHAP team at Quen Rei, 20 miles from the DMZ. The doctor was not anxious to join the team, as a MILPHAP member had been killed three weeks earlier and the staff were frequent targets of snipers. Jim was grateful for his delta assignment. Steve regaled us with descriptions of the British colony adjacent to mainland China.

I worked with Dr. Vinh to reconcile allocation of MOH funds for district health stations. Graft and theft significantly affected distribution, a practice Vinh was unable to counter. His frustration was evident as we pored over invoices of items that never arrived.

Over drinks at the officers' club, a FAC pilot related the stoic attitude of peasants during military operations. He flew shotgun over an operation near Bac Lieu, watching farmers calmly plowing fields and planting rice as airstrikes and gunships attacked nearby trees. The farmers seemed oblivious to the carnage. The situation worsened with the arrival of armored personnel carriers (APCs) carrying huge 155 mm howitzers on trailers. The guns were assembled and began firing directly over the farmers. Although the water buffalo were frightened, the unfazed farmers continued their toil. Not all such incidents had a pleasant ending as I soon learned.

I edited the monthly report and Co Ha typed the document. Her spelling led to amusing results as "disease" became "siscease," and "typhoid" was "topcold." As she typed, a multicolored bus bounced over the muddy ruts and stopped in front of the ER. When a bus arrived in this fashion, it meant one thing: casualties.

Eight patients climbed, hobbled, or were carried from the vehicle. Several were wrapped in muddy and blood-soaked blankets. All were women and children from a nearby hamlet. As we learned earlier, a shotgun pilot received ground fire from shacks near a canal and requested permission to make a rocket run. Permission was granted and rockets destroyed the shacks, producing the casualties we were now treating.

One woman had wounds of both legs. Jim and Vinh performed a below-knee amputation and debrided the other leg. Charlie and Dr. Redman operated on an 11-year-old boy with abdominal wounds. Pat, Joe Neal, and I tended to the others, mostly children, with lesser trauma. The story mirrored Cov's wild west story, and a cruel parody of the shotgun pilot's observations. After I worked on one of the kids, the boy said he was thirsty. I found a half-consumed glass of lemonade and handed it to him. He smiled and bowed politely. I wasn't particularly proud as I served him the drink.

At noon our hooch shook as if by earthquake, coupled with muffled, low-rumbling noises akin to artillery or airstrikes. I jumped up, preparing to run to the bunker, when an officer in an adjacent hooch yelled, "Skyhawk bombs—close."

Joan and the VN nurses developed a reporting system for TB cases, and Pat inaugurated APGAR scoring on maternity with Jim's help.

Named for Dr. Virginia Apgar, who developed the tool in 1952, the Apgar score is a rapid method to assess newborn viability. It ranks an infant shortly after birth on a 0–10 scale. A low score is associated with risk of death and need for immediate resuscitative measures. The simple scoring system was widely used in the United States, but the midwives were not aware of it. Although developed decades ago, the score was revalidated in 2020.

We presented the Apgar score and TB system to Vinh. As usual, he was receptive and enthusiastic, announcing, "You must advise and suggest things to us—we collaborate and learn together." Obviously pleased, he walked around the room, vigorously shaking everyone's hand.

In clinic an old Ba told our newest young interpreter she suffered from "con giun" or "con lai"—worms. Flashing a smile, the woman pulled a wiggling 8" ascaris from her sweater and deposited it on the desk. The frightened interpreter jumped out of her chair and fled to a corner of the room. Nurse Ba Phuoc calmly picked up the repulsive creature and put it in one of the shiny new COLOMBO metal waste-cans. She shared a laugh with the worm's former owner as they coaxed the young girl to her seat.

Drs. Vinh and Redman operated on two brothers with harelips. Before the procedure, Vinh drew plans for the incisions on the blackboard, explaining the French technique he used. Harelip was the most common congenital defect seen in VN, although no more prevalent than elsewhere. But in the States, plastic surgery was performed during infancy, whereas defects persisted in VN due to a lack of surgical availability. The boys were nine and 11 years old.

Vinh later visited them on the surgical ward. Their father knelt and kissed Vinh's hand. Although there was an American surgeon in Can Tho who could repair the lesions, the impact of a Vietnamese doctor performing these operations was immeasurable.

That afternoon Vinh saun-
tered into the MILPHAP office
where Jim Parker and I were
reviewing the pharmacy inven-
tory. Vinh sat down, put one foot
on my desk, and lit a large cigar.
He was in a particularly good
humor.

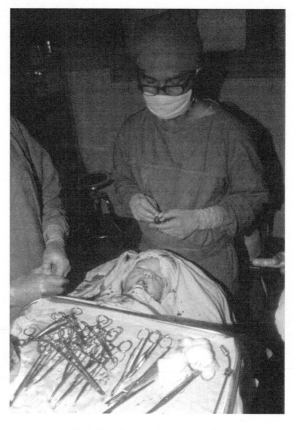

"Would you like to go to the
sea this afternoon?" He held his
hands as if aiming a rifle, "We will
shoot birds and have luncheon in
a place I know."

Charlie entered the room and
asked, "Is it safe?"

Vinh clenched the cigar
in his teeth and held his hands,
palms upward, "I don't know—I
think so—can you go?"

When Vinh answered, "I
think so," it usually meant we
would be accompanied by a cadre
of bodyguards. We nodded our
assent.

We met Vinh and his entourage at noon. In addition to

Harelip surgery by Dr. Vinh.

his Land Rover, a hospital ambulance, a jeep, and a three-quarter-ton truck were
parked on the driveway. Mrs. Vinh, Co Phung, the police chief, the public works
director, and several men carrying carbines and submachine guns were inside the
vehicles, which held additional weapons, plus picnic baskets and several bottles of
cognac.

Outside town, the caravan took a road leading to the sea, about 6 km east. After
a couple of kilometers, the road became impassable, and we transferred to sampans.
We continued on the canal for another kilometer or two, then traversed a muddy
bank on foot, ultimately arriving at a cement house decorated with Chinese lettering and fenced by wire and metal stakes. A middle-aged Chinese man emerged
and welcomed us. Nearby was a grove of lychee nut trees and several neat rows of
planted corn. Mrs. Vinh and the other women set the sumptuous picnic on blankets;
a seven-course feast, topped by cognac. Following the meal, Vinh invited us to shoot
some birds.

Several members of the party grabbed weapons and trudged through knee-deep
water to get close enough to a flock of white egrets for a shot. A policeman bagged a
bird, although retrieving the animal required wading through even deeper water. I
fired my camera. None of the MILPHAP docs took up Vinh's offer to hunt.

After a few minutes of unsuccessful hunting, the group walked to the boats for the trip to the vehicles. Such outings were popular among wealthy VN and French in earlier times but did not feature heavily armed guards and two-way radios.

Bac Lieu received another repatriate. A lad of 18 carrying an M1 carbine walked to the compound's front gate and yelled, "Chieu Hoi!" The bewildered guard wasn't clear what to do but confiscated the weapon and held the obliging young man as the sergeant of the guard was summoned. The youth could have caused considerable mischief if he had been a dedicated VC. He managed to get within 10 feet of the compound's gate with a weapon.

UCSF wrote they accepted Dr. Vinh for a three-month refresher course in surgery if the necessary permits, visas, and leave of absence could be obtained. Jim arranged the program, but the logistics would be my headache.

Another example of Dowling's predictions now faced us. The MACV colonel ordered all civilian and military personnel on loan to USAID, including MILPHAP, to live off-compound. I was disappointed but asked the USAID administrator if suitable city housing could be found for our team. Vinh told me several homes downtown might accommodate us. That afternoon we accompanied a middle-aged real estate agent to view prospective sites. The tour was depressing but enlightening.

We visited five large houses that were once elegant mansions of French or wealthy Vietnamese merchants. All were in poor repair and would require extensive renovation. Trash, graffiti, broken plumbing, peeling paint and plaster, plus vermin despoiled the once beautiful homes. Despite these drawbacks, the tour provided a glimpse of life during colonial times. The homes had features that resembled the Dalat hotel: extensive use of marble, hand-painted tiles, ornate staircases, exotic wood paneling, and multistoried elegance. However, none of the buildings was suitable. As we toured the final home, Vinh whispered it had been the residence of Tran Trinh Trach, the "Ong Lon" (great man) of the delta, whose tomb we visited a few days earlier. It was a sad ending to a once proud family. I later learned our guide was one of Trach's sons. I could not imagine his emotions as he escorted the group through his former home.

Later, Vinh and I met with contractors working on hospital projects. The meeting was frustrating: the men demanded more money than agreed and gave no excuses for delays. After one difficult interaction, Vinh walked out of the room in disgust. He patted me on the back as he offered me a Ruby Queen, advising philosophically, "In the Orient you must be patient—but not too patient. Progress is slow." We both smiled as I accepted his cigarette, but no further progress was made with the contractors.

Night call reminded me of an ER in the States—a drunken man on a bicycle hit a pothole and went over the handlebars. He sustained multiple facial and tongue lacerations with loss of several teeth. It required two hours to repair his facial and tongue wounds. Attempting to sew a constantly moving tongue is challenging. Fortunately, the local anesthetic and his alcoholic condition made the job easier.

The Bac Lieu airfield was surrounded by gunships and other war vehicles, but we managed to secure a chopper for a trip to the Vinh Chau health station. We were flying at 2,000 feet, enjoying the cool air with both side doors open. Suddenly, the starboard door gunner grabbed the microphone dangling from the ceiling and yelled into the mouthpiece. We banked sharply to port, as I struggled to hang on. I was dumbfounded, until I looked past the gunner and saw a chopper 50 yards off our starboard beam. The craft had also made visual contact and was performing an emergency turn. The evasive actions by both ships prevented an almost certain mid-air collision. No one mentioned how the near miss occurred, but we were grateful for the pilots' quick responses. The remainder of our trip was uneventful. Another example of our accident-prone environment.

American and ARVN casualties were predominately due to enemy action, but accidents such as midair collisions, friendly fire, car crashes, equipment malfunction, and other calamities caused thousands of deaths. The number and scope of such incidents are magnified in a war zone, already a deadly place. More than 10,000 U.S. deaths during the war were arbitrated to noncombatant etiologies, including diseases and accidental causes.

As we landed, we saw a group of ARVN rangers deplaning from a recent operation. From a distance they looked like children who had been playing war games, small men with oversize helmets and large backpacks. However, as we walked past the soldiers, their weathered faces, heavy with age and determination, betrayed decades-long acquaintance with war. Holes in their boots were patched with inner tubes and their uniforms showed similar repairs. This was no game.

Choppers and a small L-19 observer aircraft buzzed overhead at 5:00 a.m. in preparation for an operation near Vi Thanh. Although the hamlet was 20 km distant, the earth vibrated, and windows rattled as ordnance was expended.

On call that evening, I watched a man with advanced TB die from pulmonary hemorrhage. He coughed massive amounts of blood and choked himself to death. It was not a pleasant sight; there was little I could do other than suction some of the blood from his mouth and give sedation. Other patients on the ward, several of whom had TB, watched in horror. Most had hemoptysis, or bloody sputum, on a daily basis. I thought of Chopin, Chekhov, and Keats, as

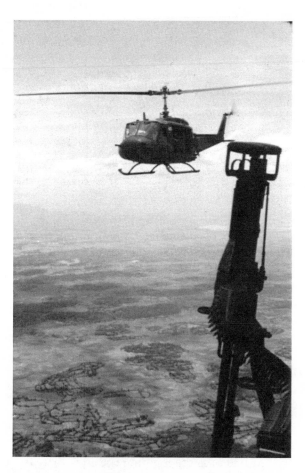

Near midair collision of gunships.

well as operatic and literary characters with consumption, and their romanticized deaths. But to witness a person drown in his own blood is a frightening and frustrating experience, even for a physician.

We were visited by Tran Van Lam, a candidate for one of the 60 Vietnamese senate seats, and a friend of Dr. Vinh. The man had an impressive résumé, including chairman of the VN bank, speaker of the house, ambassador to New Zealand-Australia, and other accolades. We met in Vinh's office as Lam campaigned across the delta. Speaking excellent English, his views reflected those of the government and he probably said what we wanted to hear. Nevertheless, it was an enlightening discussion, with a few unexpected disclosures. When asked of the French rule, Lam bluntly said France failed to realize Vietnam's nationalistic ambitions after World War II and was unable to reestablish an effective colonial government. The Viet Minh were not satisfied, and Ho Chi Minh fought and ultimately defeated the French. Lam discounted the "domino" theory if Ho had successfully managed to establish a communist Vietnam. Lam told us the country would have become an independent nation, like Yugoslavia. He concluded America backed the French too little, too late, and didn't adequately supervise the Diem regime, which could have been a model Asian democracy. Lam supported the current Saigon government and spoke optimistically of the future. Vinh listened attentively to his sunny predictions but made no comments.

Vinh held a farewell dinner for Bac Si's Stark and Redman and Pat Krebsbach, who would return to civilian nursing.

We received four gunship casualties, another variation of the aircraft-farmer story. An old peasant was livid as we amputated his thumb. Co Phung translated his commentary of rage. He and his family were in their paddy planting rice when a helicopter began firing at them. They were in the open and had no weapons. When the gunship flew above them, they did not run. As we had learned, the method to determine if a farmer is "VC" or friendly is his behavior when approached by aircraft. If he flees, he is presumed to be enemy—if he stands his ground, friendly. The farmer knew this system and continued planting. Nevertheless, the aircraft commenced firing—seriously injuring his children and killing his water buffalo. These oft-repeated scenarios were senseless.

The morning 'bou departed with our USAID nurse and the two American physicians, Redman and Stark. Nurses and midwives gave Pat a tearful parting. Many citizens of Bac Lieu owed their lives to her, and the AMA doctors had fulfilled their mission of aid.

Most of the rice paddies had been planted and the soggy land would soon blossom with a new crop. The paddies were a dull brown but would become green as the rice matured.

Bac Si Vinh was a bachelor as his wife took the children to a school in the north. He expressed anxiety of his proposed visit to America. "It will be difficult and strange for me in Hoa Ky—you must guide and show me the path." Except for a brief interval in France and vacations in the Orient, he had not left VN.

At 1:30 a.m. the officers' club was deserted except for a young 2nd Lt., sipping a Pepsi. He stared blankly as he replayed the Beatles' "We Can Work It Out." After the sixth recording, I left him to his thoughts. He was a "short timer" and had only a few weeks in country. I thought of Dowling's predictions and the soldier's future psychological troubles.

I flew to Saigon to obtain a passport for my leave in Hong Kong. Life in the capital bustled, but the mood was anxious. The September election and the threat of renewed terrorist attacks worried the populace.

The city was plastered with candidates' posters. As I wandered through Saigon, I had forgotten how hectic it had become. Black market items of all descriptions were sold on sidewalks, as hawkers and pimps yelled at pedestrians, enticing them to buy, or enter a bar: "Come inside Joe, I show you good time."

I met Drs. Stark and Redman at the Rex hotel for drinks, along with other AMA physicians preparing to leave country. One was Dr. P, an Ob-Gyn doctor from New Jersey who had worked with a MILPHAP team in the central highlands. He sipped his Scotch and speculated, "I'll be on the outside looking in when I return to the States—have you ever heard of a Jesuit doing a tubal ligation?"

He continued, "We worked at Pat Smith's hospital in Montagnard country. One day the midwives called me for a native woman in labor with a central placenta previa who was bleeding badly. We took her into surgery and did a traditional C-section. We got the baby out OK, but as we were closing, I turned to Pat and said, 'You know, there's something we need to do, no matter what our church tells us— we've got to tie that woman's tubes'."

He leaned forward and ran his fingers through his hair. "Now, I'm a Jesuit, and in two years, I will be a priest, God willing. But I'm also a physician. It would be criminal to let that woman leave the hospital to become pregnant again. She lives 50 km from the hospital in a remote hamlet and has no way of understanding the risk of uterine rupture with another pregnancy. I had no choice: I tied her tubes. They may nail me to the cross when I return, but I feel I made the right decision."

Placenta previa, or low-lying placenta near or at the mouth of the cervix, is a common cause of bleeding during the latter phases of pregnancy, and a major cause of fetal and maternal mortality. When severe, treatment includes emergency C-section. A subsequent pregnancy with attempted vaginal delivery risks uterine rupture. Thus, the dictum—once a C-section, always a caesarean. This policy dominated obstetrical practice for nearly 60 years, and in 1974, nearly 99 percent of women with a prior C-section delivered via a repeat operation. Even today as elective C-sections are commonplace, subsequent vaginal delivery should include facilities for emergency surgery. Dr. P knew it would be impossible for this woman to have a repeat C-section as she could die of a ruptured uterus. Despite his religious beliefs, he sterilized the woman.

Redman raised his glass, suggesting he run for Pope on the "sterilization ticket." "Hell, all us protestants will vote for you," he voiced as the group smiled and finished their drinks.

Dr. Merritt Stark departed for the United States following two months in Bac Lieu, but his ultimate Vietnam experience consumed many years. He graduated from the University of Colorado School of Medicine, trained at Yale, the Cleveland Clinic, and Rochester, New York, and was a practicing Colorado pediatrician in 1967 when he volunteered for the AMA program. After his Bac Lieu tenure, he returned to Vietnam in 1969 as a public health official, remaining until the fall of Saigon in 1975. In addition to his marine son, he had five other children, several of whom were involved in Vietnam humanitarian efforts. One daughter died tragically in a crash of an Operation Baby Lift flight to ferry orphan children to America. Stark later served as medical director of an Indian Health Service in South Dakota (Merritt Stark, MD, 1916–1996).

Tan Son Nhut at dawn—buttermilk sky and the Eighth Aerial Port where 200 soldiers awaited flights throughout VN, and I to Bac Lieu. The port had been enlarged since my arrival months earlier, although it remained dirty and disorganized. A large sign in the center of the building proclaimed: *NO SLEEPING IN THE PORT OVERNIGHT*.

Flight 440 was eventually called, and I boarded the Caribou with officers wearing freshly minted tropical fatigues who dragged their bags across the tarmac to the aircraft.

The crew chief, recognizing new arrivals, gave a colorful introduction of flying over enemy territory: "All right gentlemen—this is flight 440 bound for Can Tho, Vinh Long, Soc Trang, and Bac Lieu. Listen up, 'cause I'm only going to say this once. Our first stop is Vinh Long. Please observe the fasten seat belt sign and the no smoking lamp. Once we're airborne I'll put out the light and you can smoke. When we descend, it will be lit again. We'll have a nice soft touchdown at Vinh Long for you." He snickered as he glanced at the pilot, who winked. The chief added, "If for any reason we need to make an emergency landing, you'll hear six alarm blasts. Check your seat belts—all loose articles as well as your weapons. Take everything out of your pockets—we don't want any pencil or pen stabbings. Again, fasten your seat belts and cross your arms on the back of the person in front of you. When the plane comes to a stop, proceed to the rear of the plane—provided this thing is still in one piece. Any questions?" He added, "Oh, by the way, if you have any problems, or get sick—use your helmet. That stuff smells up the plane something fierce." With those parting remarks, he retreated to the cockpit as the plane increased speed for takeoff.

The flight was uneventful, and the new officers appreciated the absence of excitement. All passengers save me had deplaned prior to Bac Lieu, the last stop.

That afternoon I met our new AMA volunteer physician, Dr. Pio Pezzi, a surgeon from Pennsylvania. Originally from Rome, Pezzi was the product of an illustrious Italian family. A tall, bespectacled, kindly man, Pio completed medical school in Rome, followed by surgical training in Pennsylvania. Friendly, outgoing, and articulate, he had no illusions about the challenges he would face. Dr. Vinh was very pleased to have another surgical colleague, a gift from USAID, which provided a continuous supply of AMA physicians.

The chief Saigon midwife visited to discuss the loop clinic. She acknowledged resistance to the program at MOH, but Jim convinced her the clinic was a pilot project. We were elated when he approved the program, but recommended a hiatus during the upcoming elections. Although noncommittal for the future, we cautiously continued inserting IUD's.

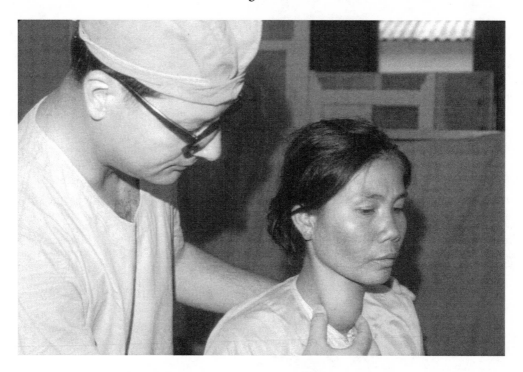

Dr. Pio Pezzi examining patient with thyroid mass.

ARVN forces totaling more than 2,000 converged on a site near Vi Tranh for a large operation. Despite reports of massive numbers of the enemy, few were engaged, a typical scenario. As usual, the VC's intelligence exceeded ours.

On another front, Jim and I listened to radio dispatches at the CP bunker from besieged Green Berets at Hai Yen, a subsector near Ca Mau. The calm voice of a captain was chilling as he described attacks on his position. Mortars, recoilless rifles, and machine guns had zeroed in on his troops, with shells falling within yards of his position. In a matter-of-fact tone, he described the situation and gave the enemy's coordinates. Fortunately, choppers returning from another operation were diverted and rescued the embattled group. The VC retreated into the countryside and no American or ARVN troops were injured, although the outpost was heavily damaged. The officer's performance was an impressive display of military professionalism under fire.

Jim spent several hours caring for a woman attacked by thieves. They assaulted and robbed her of the family's funds from planting rice, leaving her to die on the road. She had multiple injuries requiring surgery. The assailants were unknown, but not VC—merely brigands.

Our former interpreter, Co Tuyet, was brought to the ER by her family. Her condition was shocking. Two months had elapsed since we dismissed her for inappropriate and bizarre behavior. We had suggested her parents take her to a psychiatric facility in Saigon, but she was kept at home and given Chinese medicine. Her appearance alarmed us—pale, thin, unkempt, with incoherent mumbling. There were signs of physical illness—paralysis of one eye and muscles on her left side. We suspected a brain tumor or infection and arranged transport to Saigon. It was a sad commentary for this once smiling teenager.

Bac Lieu was again placed on high alert with a 6:00 p.m. curfew. It was the eve of a VC holiday that dated to the French era, roughly translated as "Hate Foreigners." The evening's 105 mm howitzer bombardment was especially heavy, including many "charge 7" shells. As elections neared, Vinh was visibly anxious and predicted voting irregularities and renewed VC activity.

Thanks to USAID, some sections of the concrete hospital driveway had been poured. For nearly a year a local public works official had refused Dr. Vinh's requests to pave the muddy, rutted access. The man also objected to use of USAID funding or Chieu Hoi labor. Vinh was ecstatic, and spent both days supervising the 50-odd workers. Unfortunately, the project was abruptly halted and Mr. Mowatt told to withhold further USAID support. We had a road to nowhere, but at least part of the driveway was paved. It wasn't clear who ordered the work stoppage. A disconsolate Vinh was forced to seek other support to complete the job.

The 15th day of the 7th Chinese lunar month is the traditional date to honor ancestors. The celebration resembles the Mexican holiday "Día de Muertos," the Day of the Dead. Imitation money akin to Chinese joss paper, together with paper dolls and clothing fashioned from paper, are burned, as rice and other foods are offered to the departed spirits to gain access to heaven. The Vietnamese celebration is called "Cung Co Hon," and small fires of offerings were visible in front of many Bac Lieu homes and businesses.

I was witness to a variety of Bac Lieu vignettes. Many were puzzles. Our quarters were cleaned by "hooch girls," who chattered like chipmunks as they polished boots, made beds, carried trash, and swept floors. Their day began at 8:00 a.m. as they displayed their badges to enter the compound. The women usually completed hooch duties by 10:30 a.m., followed by cleaning latrine, and mowing grass. Whenever a senior officer approached, they worked furiously, but by mid-afternoon they could be found in a hooch, resting beneath a fan. Occasionally, a worker would be suspected of theft or being a VC sympathizer, and dismissed. I recalled the woman who detonated the mine downtown. But most girls were honest and loyal. In fact, many were ARVN widows or wives. Our girl, Ba Hai, was paid 3,000 piastres a month, plus tips. She was 32 years of age and had five children; three had been killed by a VC bomb. A year earlier her ARVN husband was abducted by the VC near Dalat and his fate was unknown. Despite these hardships, she smiled and attended her duties while softly humming. She socialized with the other hooch girls and giggled at the slightest comment by an officer. How did she retain her sunny attitude?

An F-19 plane had a narrow escape. The pilot completed a pass marking enemy positions for a F104 jet, as he saw tracers coursing toward his craft. The tiny craft shuddered as several machine gun slugs hit one wing and the engine cowling. One bullet punctured the oil cooling system with a sudden increase in engine temperature and loss of power. The F104 flew "shotgun" for the F-19 as the little plane limped toward Bac Lieu's field. The pilot feared the engine would freeze at any moment. A second F-19 was dispatched to help chaperone the damaged craft, which made it safely to base.

Another AMA physician joined the team: Dr. Rudolf Toch, a pediatrician from Massachusetts, although born in Germany. He was a faculty member in pediatric oncology at Harvard and a respected physician. Toch had a squarish face, modest height, and a thick shock of hair with a dark, bushy moustache. Confident, affable, with a positive attitude, he proved to be a great asset to the pediatric service. At the time, we were not aware of his many accomplishments. Toch always had a supply of balloons for kids on Pediatrics, and words of wisdom for Joe Neal.

Bac Si Lui, a senior MOH physician, flew from Saigon to meet us. He was a flamboyant individual, sporting army fatigues and combat boots, and accompanied by a bodyguard brandishing a Czech automatic rifle. The inquisitive doctor was very receptive to the loop clinic and approved the project on the spot, an official decision we had awaited for months,

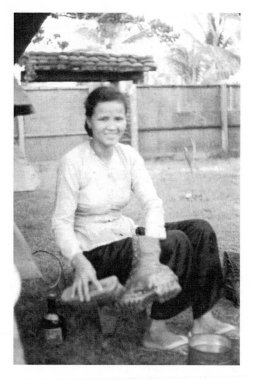

Hooch girl cleaning boots.

and allied with the recent announcement of the chief midwife. Lui also said the clinic could continue uninterrupted during the elections. Jim suggested the clinic was the most important contribution of our MILPHAP team—doctor Lui agreed. After Lui departed, Jim confided he wasn't certain Lui had the authority to approve the clinic, but we would accept his decision. I agreed.

That afternoon Vinh invited me to a city council meeting to discuss the driveway project. Council members and the province chief expressed encouragement, although the villain was the public works director, who was not present. Vinh was popular with city leaders. I never understood why the public works director opposed him. Local politics is often personal. Meanwhile, the project awaited funding, which was not awarded at the council meeting: Vinh's dilemma had yet to be solved.

Arriving suddenly and with terrific power, a wind of gale force swept through Bac Lieu with torrential rain. Monsoon gusts of 60 mph blew through hooches and flooded walkways. Power was lost in the compound as lightning flashes illuminated the darkness. Several trees were felled, and a pending military operation was aborted. Hospital activities were similarly curtailed, although a few braved the torment to attend clinic.

Joe Neal and Steve Reynard were short timers. On return to America, Steve would be discharged from the army to complete training at the LA County Hospital. Joe would advance to third year at Stanford medical school. Dr. Toch suggested Joe should be made a senior, having managed diseases his professors had only read about in textbooks.

For three days weather precluded any military operations. Several choppers took off, only to return, buffeted by wind and rain. Three aircraft crashed at Vinh Long, killing one pilot—more "civilian" wartime accidents.

Hospital clinics remained slow, but the wards were full. In fact, it was difficult to discharge patients from the relative comfort and dryness of the wards. One old man was discharged, only to show up in clinic an hour later, demanding readmission.

The war was accelerating, and the September elections provided an opportunity for terrorist attacks. MACV intelligence (G-2) officers scrambled to ascertain intentions of the enemy. The VC could attack and disrupt the populace at will, frustrating the efforts of my MACV colleagues, as we learned that afternoon.

A young intelligence officer read from a notepad of the recent shelling in Soc Trang, briefing the colonel and assembled officers: "At 11:00 a.m. the Soc Trang airfield was attacked with 75 mm recoilless rifles. Gunships were dispatched and returned fire." He cleared his throat and continued, "The attack was believed to be a diversionary measure to commit helicopter support to Soc Trang, as Can Tho was then attacked from six separate positions by recoilless rifles and mortars. Eight rounds hit the MACV compound and the ARVN hospital, destroying several wards. Other projectiles landed throughout the city, including the marketplace."

The colonel interrupted and asked if fire had been returned. The lieutenant responded, "No sir, helicopters were airborne in such a short time the 105s couldn't fire without calling off the gunships."

"Damn. As we feared," snapped the colonel. "Big cities are hit and what happens? People lose morale and voting will be inhibited."

I nodded in agreement as he continued, "This is a battle for the will of the populace—VC attack and intimidate residents, disrupting voting. How can a fair election proceed under these conditions?" The colonel's ire was evident as he acknowledged how easily the VC could attack with demoralizing effects on national elections. Frustrated and angered, the colonel abruptly ended the briefing. As I left the room an aide informed me the move of the MILPHAP team to the city had been cancelled. I breathed a sigh of relief; at least there was some good news. None of our group wished to abandon the compound's security.

Can Tho was attacked and General Minh increased security around Bac Lieu in anticipation of local VC activity. Lightships were aloft and artillery salvos persisted until dawn.

I had a twinge of guilt as Bac Lieu prepared for a possible attack, but happily boarded a 'bou for Saigon and my visit to Hong Kong. The capital was bracing for violence and a curfew was in effect throughout the city. The country held its breath. But Saigon's suspenseful mood was masked by beautiful flower markets downtown.

Chapter Sources

Sven Cnattingius, Stefan Johansson, and Neda Razaz. "Apgar Score and Risk of Neonatal Death Among Preterm Infants." *New England Journal of Medicine* 383, no. 1 (2020): 49–57.

Merritt W. Stark. *Special Collection and Archives*. University of Colorado, Boulder.

Bruce Cohen and Meredith Atkins. "A Brief History of Vaginal Birth After Caesarian Section. *Clinical Obstetrics and Gynecology* 44, no. 3 (2001): 604–8.

14

September

Paving the Future, Reflections

I returned from a week of Hong Kong's fast-paced life in the shadow of Red China to the soggy paddies of Bac Lieu. A bomb threat at my hotel was a reminder the Red Chinese dragon was near, although my vacation was otherwise pleasant, with excellent food, sightseeing, and purchase of tailor-made suits fashioned within 24 hours.

The hospital was unchanged. No attacks occurred in Bac Lieu during the national elections, although Gia Rai and Phuoc Long were mortared. Can Tho's shelling was documented in a *Time* magazine article that listed 46 fatalities, but I learned the death toll was considerably greater. Bac Lieu was not attacked, but the hospital received many casualties, including one from within its walls. A gunfight between two drunken ARVNs led to the death of a boy in the line of fire, the son of one of the soldiers. A court martial would decide the fate of the assailant.

Doctor Vinh remained focused on the paving project, but work remained stalled. Undaunted, he vowed to form a citizen's committee to finance the project.

Although the VC attacked other provincial hospitals, our facility remained neutral territory and treated several VC, and their medics referred patients to the ER. Jim was the recipient of direct attention, called to treat the wife of a VC colonel. The woman arrived on the eve of the election and her husband instructed the midwives to summon Bac Si Jones. They were reluctant, but the officer insisted. The woman was postpartum and critically ill with septic shock. The VC colonel and his lieutenants kept a watchful eye as Jim attended her. The situation was precarious, and the midwives feared for Jim's safety. The struggle to save the woman's life persisted for several days.

The election was reported as fair, but Vinh and Jim observed many irregularities at polling sites. Each presidential candidate was listed on a separate sheet of paper. The voter was to drop his or her selection in the ballot box. But papers of the other candidates were not collected and could have been deposited separately. Several peace candidates were elected, and it wasn't clear if the VC influenced their election. Violence was reported, but the national election proceeded without major incidents and more than 80 percent of eligible voters participated. The newly elected National Constituent Assembly promptly framed and adopted a new anticommunist constitution and ratified Thieu's presidency. Some observers believed Vietnam's road to democracy was enhanced, but there was little change in governmental policy and rampant corruption continued as prosecution of the war was increasingly waged by the United States. The election was a lost opportunity—perhaps the last.

In Bac Lieu, statistics often belied the facts. Determining accurate birth rates and perinatal mortality were goals of Jim's maternity program. But an incident made Jim wonder if he could ever collect meaningful data.

Jim and the chief midwife, Ba Thao, conducted their routine rounds on the postpartum ward, the Ba mechanically uttering the words "accouchement normal" as they passed from bed to bed. At the last three beds Ba Thao exclaimed, "All normal deliveries, Bac Si." She began to leave when Jim caught sight of a mother in the last bed. He stopped and addressed Ba Thao as he pointed to the woman, "Wait a minute, didn't she have a premature delivery? I remember the mole on her cheek, and her baby couldn't have been a thousand grams.... What happened to the baby?"

Ba Thao looked at her notebook, awoke the mother, and quickly asked several questions in Vietnamese. She turned to Jim, "Oh yes," Ba Thao replied. "She had a small baby, but it died. She wanted a child, so she bought one from the girl in the next bed. It is very common."

Jim couldn't believe what he heard—something from a bad novel. "But what about the mother?" he asked. "Oh, she went home. She didn't want her baby anyway," Ba Thao said offhandedly.

Thus, one baby dies, and another is exchanged by a mother who is not listed as pregnant, and the dead premature infant is not recorded in the census. This was routine for the midwives, but a statistical nightmare.

The VC colonel's wife slowly improved under Jim's management. The husband didn't visit during the day, but I frequently saw him during evening rounds on the maternity ward. He and his colleagues eyed me carefully but made no threatening gestures as I performed my duties.

The MACV commanding colonel called all personnel for a special briefing. Rumors had circulated of an invasion of North Vietnam. "Please stand for the senior advisor," barked a major who preceded the colonel into the room. "Gentlemen, be seated." he ordered, as he strode to the podium next to the movie projector. "I have not called you here to chew you out, but I'll do so if you don't heed my comments." He continued in an authoritative voice, "The following was received from MACV Headquarters this morning. I'll read it without comment, as it is self-explanatory." The statement told of a new electronic barrier under construction at the DMZ. The barrier was to be completed by early 1968 and would make it "increasingly difficult" for supplies or personnel to infiltrate from North Vietnam. The notice warned American personnel not to discuss the project. The colonel finished the reading, rolled up the paper, and stuffed it in his trouser pocket, asking, "Any questions, gentlemen?" No one responded. Apparently satisfied, he nodded and walked stiffly out of the room. The U.S. government was placing emphasis on the electronic project, but feared security leaks. At least we had not invaded North Vietnam.

McNamara's line, "The Barrier System," was a fortified project on the northern border of Vietnam at the DMZ from the South China sea west to Laos. It included high tech electronic systems to detect movement of North Vietnamese troops or equipment as well as mines and other weapon systems to interdict intrusion from the north. The project was controversial and expensive but pushed forward by Secretary McNamara at the highest levels of government. The secrecy alluded to in the colonel's briefing was short-lived, and terms such as "McNamara's Wall" were quickly adopted by the press. After the 1968 Tet offensive and the bloody battle of Khe Sanh at the DMZ, construction was halted.

Hospital routine was affected by the return of hot, drier weather, which lowered census. The summer monsoon was ebbing. Vinh was depressed as he wandered through the hospital. He was watching workmen pour cement for the roof of the new clinic as I approached. "Chao Bac Si," I said as we met. He smiled and limply shook my hand, pointing with his other to the fortified roof, "Very good, very strong. We can use as bomb shelter." He asked of my Hong Kong trip and I mentioned some of the attractions, which improved his attitude. But his conversation quickly drifted to the unfinished driveway and lack of financial support. With a gentle wave, he shuffled to his office.

Police brought a VC to the ER under heavy guard, although security was unnecessary. He was wounded by a claymore mine a week earlier and had been treated in jail. But for two days he would not eat. True enough, he couldn't open his mouth—his jaws were tightly clenched: tetanus. By noon the fellow was so rigid he could not have crawled, much less walked to freedom. Observing his status, guards abandoned the young man on the ward as we struggled to provide adequate sedation and address his labored breathing.

The ARVN compound noon bell sounded, and I headed to lunch across the

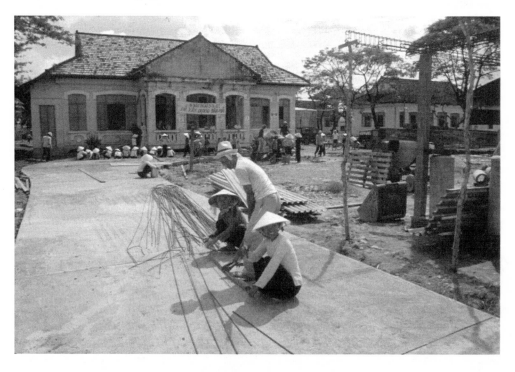

Paving the hospital driveway.

unfinished cement driveway. Before I reached the MACV back gate, Co Phung ran to me, calling, "Bac Si, Bac Si—wounds!"

A 30-year-old woman lay on the exam table with mortar fragments in her back, chest, and left arm. Joan poked her head in the emergency room door asking, "Anything I can do?"

Joan's help was welcome, and we spent the next 30 minutes cleaning and suturing injuries. As we finished, the woman calmly sat up and walked to a bed in the adjacent room. She had not shown any emotion or signs of pain, impressive stoicism.

Lunch was further delayed as an ARVN ambulance bounced through the gate, stopping at the ER steps. A crowd formed as the staff unloaded two patients. Earlier that morning a loud explosion was heard near Gia Rai. ARVN soldiers found a young woman and a boy in a roadside ditch, covered with dirt and the remnants of a homemade bomb. The boy's legs were amputated plus he had multiple shrapnel wounds. The young woman was more fortunate but sustained serious injuries. They had planned to bury the bomb in the road, but it detonated prematurely. Transport to the hospital required several hours.

Joan and I worked on the boy, who had the most life-threatening wounds. Despite his injuries, he was awake and looked at us with hate and terror. We cleaned and dressed his wounds and gave IV fluids and antibiotics. Vinh and Pezzi modified the amputations, and operated on the woman. Both victims remained critically ill.

As I returned to my hooch, a captain approached me on the boardwalk. He had consumed a few beers and was wearing a pair of Bermuda shorts, flip-flops, and a T-shirt bearing the name of a major university. He began, "Say, I hear you've got the two VC from Gia Rai who blew themselves up." I nodded as he asked, "How bad are they hurt?" I said the boy is likely to die but the woman will probably recover. He took a long pull from a can of beer and responded, "Good, that's what he deserves— God damn terrorists! I don't care if one is a kid—these damn people should all be shot."

I opened the door to my hooch, but the officer grabbed my arm, "Can you release them tomorrow? We could really cook up a good psy-war effort in Gia Rai. It's times like this we can magnify hate for the VC—when it's fresh in their minds. You know, just like the old lynch mobs. Boy, this could really be great."

Not believing what I heard, I told him the pair were in no condition to be moved. He snarled, "Hell, I don't give a damn if they die anyway—think of how much good this would do—especially if they can confess."

I finally convinced the officer I could not release the patients, but he insisted it would make a great spectacle. After a few moments he tired of the discussion and walked to the officers' club.

The incident was an example of behavior exhibited by some MACV officers, reminiscent of the drunken singers. But murder of women or children, even if terrorists, was beyond the pale for most officers.

Hot weather alternated with intermittent rain. Showering helped, but humidity and sweat soon engulfed one's clothing. The heat seemed to attract patients. There was an overflow in the ER and a baby was abandoned on the steps of the maternity ward. Despite our efforts, it died a few hours later. Dr. Toch estimated it to be one week old. Meanwhile, the VC colonel's wife slowly improved and her departure was anticipated.

Miraculously, the injured boy improved. Patients in the ward were unaffected by the presence of guards and paid little attention to the boy. As his guards dozed in the afternoon heat, the boy played with a toy furnished by Co Anh. Kids showed remarkable resilience despite often horrific injuries or illness.

A smaller than normal clinic greeted me, and I thought, "Maybe this will be a quiet day." But what began innocently enough developed into a hellish series of events.

I was writing a script for TB meds when the ER called. The interpreter calmly said, "Bac Si, we have a patient

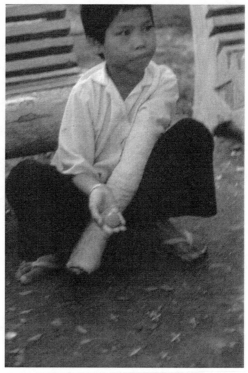

Girl injured by VC playing jacks.

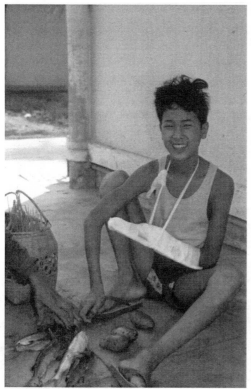

Injured boy with fish caught in canal.

for you." A 20-year-old with a fever of 104 degrees lay on the ER examining table. She was seizing and coughing thick sputum. She had been sick for three weeks and developed convulsions today. I observed a "blown pupil" (dilated pupil), suggesting localized brain pathology as well as paralysis and a stiff neck. The staff set up a lumbar puncture (spinal tap). Exam of the fluid didn't reveal signs of meningitis, but we gave fluids and antibiotics. She died a few hours later without a diagnosis. Throughout the ordeal her family poured Chinese medicine down her throat as I silently cursed our primitive facilities.

I was again called to the ER for three casualties from Gia Rai. The first two were a young woman and her eight-year-old daughter who had been hit by a mortar. Both had fragment wounds. Dr. Pezzi immediately took the girl to surgery.

The third patient was a young Cambodian man believed to be a VC. He was bleeding from several superficial lacerations and covered with mud as he was unloaded from a cart. He had the physique of a wrestler but moaned in agony despite what appeared to be minor wounds. I asked Joan to clean the affected areas and call me when he was ready for debridement. I had no sooner returned to the clinic when Joan poked her head over the Dutch doors and said, "Dick, you'd better have another look at this guy—he's smoking."

The two recent kids with phosphorus burns died within 24 hours. Jim and Vinh picked molten pieces of metal from the bodies as wisps of acrid, white smoke rose from the surgical drapes. Jim sustained burns of his hands during the procedure. Today's patient was the unlucky recipient of a 105 mm howitzer shell loaded with white phosphorus. The ignited material continues to burn and eat its way through flesh and bone. Copper sulfate solution can neutralize the burning phosphorus, but the solution is poisonous, and only small amounts can be applied. We removed nearly 40 smoking fragments and dabbed the wounds with the copper solution, followed by soapy water. The man experienced severe pain. Despite local anesthesia and opiates, he moaned and writhed throughout the procedure.

White phosphorus is used in incendiary munitions, tracers, and smoke bombs. It continues to burn unless deprived of oxygen or chemically neutralized. Systemic phosphorus toxicity is another risk, as well as lung damage from fumes. Human

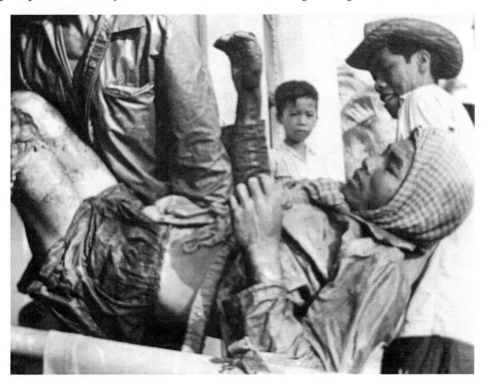

Unloading VC white phosphorus victim of a 105 mm howitzer.

rights groups have urged a multinational ban on white phosphorus weapons, but their use continues in the Middle East and elsewhere.

It mattered little if the man was a VC or innocent hamlet resident: no one should be a victim of such a fiendish weapon. We employed many terrible agents of war in VN—among the worst were phosphorus and napalm. I thought of U.S. public opinion. People berated hippies who grew beards, wore flowers, and experimented with LSD. Meanwhile, we were fighting the "holy" war, killing and maiming with hideous toys of war.

As a reward for a long day, Dr. Vinh took the doctors to a Chinese restaurant. Pezzi was convinced the establishment was the source of local cholera epidemics but promised to sample the food. Several chickens were chased from under our table as the manager dispersed inquisitive children. Vinh ordered. The first course arrived and Pezzi exclaimed in delight, "Spaghetti!" Yes, well, at least noodles, which legend held Marco Polo brought from Asia. The noodles were delicious, as were fish, duck, shrimp, and the Italian wine Pezzi provided. A cigar and café-au-lait completed our feast. We harbored fears of subsequent gastrointestinal complications, but the meal was delightful. Pezzi was developing bonds with Vinh as had his predecessors. It was a pleasant interlude.

A Green Beret lieutenant from an adjacent hooch departed at midnight for a secret mission. He and a small group of ARVN soldiers were dropped by chopper deep in the U Minh forest. They would rendezvous for pickup two days hence. Their job was to locate VC units and report their movement. This was dangerous business, with risk of capture or worse. The brave officer had graduated from

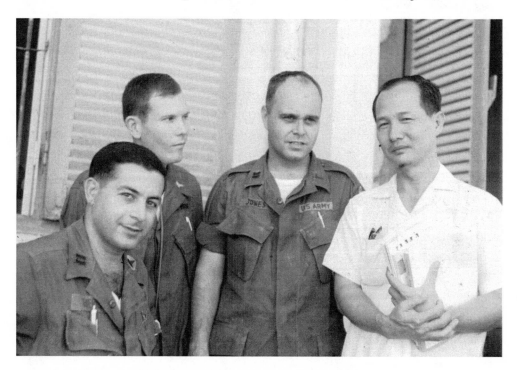

Bac Lieu doctors: Charlie Gueriera, author, Jim Jones, and Dr. Vinh.

Ranger school and was a specialist in guerrilla warfare, but I did not wish to be in his boots.

The Cambodian man with phosphorus burns died from progressive heart failure from phosphorus toxicity or the copper sulfate.

Jim left for R&R. Pezzi, Charlie, and I walked downtown to view the Bac Lieu market. We saw fruits and vegetables, several of which we couldn't identify, as well as fish, including a large barracuda, several sharks, a ray, and a trigger fish. Other sea bounty were shrimp, crabs, and eels. The seafood was unloaded onto cement tables where women rapidly cleaned the catch with large knives and cleavers. Elsewhere men pushed carts with squealing pigs. Chickens and ducks cackled from within reed baskets. My colleagues remained to watch a hog butchered, but I returned to the compound, had a beer, showered, and tried to get some rest before night call.

For months I had been told of canal blocks and the difficulties to successfully destroy and control them. Nevertheless, Gen. Minh planned a 21st divisional operation to disable and occupy a nearby block. An ARVN engineering group and a large cadre of troops were airlifted to the location. The block was destroyed by high explosives, followed by a ground assault. A MACV captain with the advancing ARVN soldiers suddenly heard an explosion and felt a searing pain in his jaw. He dropped to the ground as he grabbed his face. A soldier had tripped a wire, detonating a claymore mine. Although his wound was painful, it was superficial, and the officer continued to direct his men. The VC retreated, but were displeased, firing at choppers throughout the day. A door gunner with a machine gun wound was evacuated to the airport. I removed the bullet from his leg and he resumed to helicopter duty. The officer's facial injury was not serious. I sutured the lesion and he also returned to the ongoing battle.

Several civilian victims of the canal operation were brought to the hospital. One was a young girl with a wound from a Huey machine gun. Charlie kept the slug as a grisly souvenir. We speculated how long the VC would wait before attempting to retake the block.

September 18 was "Le Trung Thu," or "Children's Day," an event celebrated throughout the Orient, with gifts for children and the elderly. The Red Cross provided pencil sets for kids, plus food, clothing, and items for inhabitants of "old house" on hospital grounds. Most of the residents had TB, leprosy, or other chronic illnesses and were frequent visitors to the clinics. Mrs. Vinh, Charlie, and I walked through the foul-smelling building, distributing gifts to the elders who sat on their beds, clasping their hands in thanks. There were small bundles under the beds, containing the worldly possessions of these adult orphans. The head of some bedframes bore a small cross or Buddhist shrine. In one bed a blind man held the frame as his wife, also blind, extended her hands for the parcel. After receipt they placed their palms together in subservience. We were all affected by the scene and wondered what could be done for these wretched souls. The country was at war and the population suffering. Nearly one-half of children would not reach adulthood and life expectancy was low. These elderly individuals lived in the backwater and were ignored. Vinh provided them a home and food on hospital grounds, but they lived a miserable, short life. I was moved by their plight, and Mrs. Vinh was crying as we left. We returned, sobered and depressed, despite the presumed joyous occasion. Charlie later told me five children died on the pediatric ward overnight.

More casualties arrived that evening as Charlie prepared to accompany MACV on an operation in the morning. He had been assigned Steve's job until a replacement arrived.

I was occupied in the ER. An old man was hit by a homemade VC mine filled with pieces of heavy wire. I removed at least 30 one-inch sections from his arms, legs, and back, locating them with the fluoroscope, sweating under the heavy lead apron. A full moon rose, or "dem thu trang," literally, the autumn's bright moon. I was again called to operate. This time I assisted Vinh for a young boy shot in the chest. The bullet passed from the right chest through the diaphragm and into the abdomen. The boy's parents and I each donated a unit of blood. We lay on the ER tables as hospital workers performed the venipunctures, gently agitating the citrated bags to prevent clotting as the plastic containers accepted the precious red liquid.

I returned to the compound from call at 4:30 a.m. as a sleepy-eyed Charlie stumbled out of his hooch for a day of war. Within an hour, choppers were airborne. The activity was light but marred by a freak accident. An ARVN soldier walked directly into the path of a Huey tail rotor. Amazingly, despite severe lacerations the man was not killed.

As predicted, the liberated canal block was brazenly retaken by the VC, who rebuilt it in broad daylight and established regional control. Civilians were conscripted for construction. A FAC airplane flying overhead received several machine gun rounds as a token of their enmity. The VC's domination of these blocks was tenacious, reflecting their economic importance.

We received a report of plague in a nearby hamlet. Vinh and I drove to the village and sat in the village chief's house as Vinh interrogated him. Apparently three patients suffered from a "strange malady" that had taken two lives. As Vinh posed his questions, it was clear the illness resembled pneumonia, not plague. After a few minutes Vinh gave a grunt, rose, and indicated the interview had concluded. He asked me to examine the patients. The first was a middle-aged woman with cough and fever. She had pneumonia. The next was a 10-month-old infant with worms and diarrhea. The final patient was an elderly gentleman too ill to walk with advanced TB. As I listened to his lungs, he stuffed a yellow piece of paper with Chinese characters into his mouth. These tokens were to exorcise the bad spirits and bring good luck. His wife approached and began to acupuncture his neck and chest. Vinh asked for the patients to be transferred to the hospital, but a villager came forward and warned, "If they leave, the wind will enter their bodies; they will become more ill and die." Vinh threw up his hands in desperation, berated those present for their superstitions, and stormed out of the house. As we drove to Bac Lieu he calmed somewhat, but declared, "These people live in the past. Maybe the colonel thinks he can cure them with MEDCAPS, but spiritualism dies slowly. The charlatans are strong." This was the first time I'd seen Vinh rail against the MEDCAP clinics.

Bob Brittis, a pediatrician, first-generation New York Italian American, and my replacement as MOC, arrived on the morning 'bou. Tired, depressed, and alarmed by Saigon briefings, he collapsed on Jim's bed until mid-afternoon, when we gave him a brief tour of the hospital. He was even more despondent after viewing the facility.

Charlie remained in the field. The VC fared better than ARVN. The number of killed and wounded for each side was equal, and the few prisoners and captured weapons came at high cost. One MACV officer described a radio transmission as utter confusion, with choppers twirling in the sky, firing seemingly at random. One interchange went, "Hello Red Leader, this is Bravo One. Would you please inform Tiger 5 [a gunship] he is firing on us!" Fortunately, no MACV were injured, but a mistaken airstrike on ARVN soldiers killed 12 men. Later, 75 sampans were seen moving out of the area. Gunships and airplanes were called, and their awesome firepower was ready to be unleashed when it was learned the boats' cargo was fleeing civilians. The war's confusion and lethal mistakes were endless.

Doctor Vinh held a farewell party for two of our enlisted men, Sgts. Andy and Hill. The occasion provided the first meeting with Bob Brittis. Vinh gave him a warm welcome. Bob remained apprehensive about the country, and especially the food. He was shocked when offered a drink with ice, plus cookies and fresh fruits.

Our USAID nurses were leaving. Linda and Joan would soon be transferred to other hospitals and Mariana to a public health clinic near Saigon.

There were 76 USAID nurses in VN during 1967, among a total of 197 USAID health workers. Two-thirds of RNs were engaged in clinical services, predominantly in provincial MILPHAP hospitals. We were lucky to have four dedicated women assigned to Bac Lieu for most of the year. USAID nurses rendered important service but represented a small portion of nurses in Vietnam. Army and Navy RNs staffed the many military facilities. There were more than 900 army nurses in VN during 1969, and military RNs were often deployed to combat zones where they endured attacks. One army nurse, Lt. Sharon Lane, was killed by enemy action in Chu Lai. When not on duty, army and navy nurses volunteered to assist civilians, together with military physicians and corpsmen.

The pharmacy was utterly confused. Supplies had not been reordered and we had no penicillin, Demerol, or suture material. I apologized for these and other problems as I escorted Bob through the hospital.

That evening Vinh operated on two patients from his private practice. The first was a boy with a ruptured appendix who squatted atop the operating table as the OR was readied. The next was a Cambodian woman with eleven children who presented with complications of pregnancy. The product was a dead baby and a Couvelaire uterus, or abruption (rupture-detachment of the placenta). Luckily, she survived, as abruption is one of the most devastating obstetrical complications. The family could not afford blood and Joan donated a unit. As he finished surgery Vinh offered these comments, "In Vietnam a man's life is worth 5,000 piastres. They say the old, 'Ve Tay Phuong,' or 'pass to the west'; but the young also die if they cannot afford medicine." I looked at Bob Brittis who was standing behind me. He was incredulous.

The MACV compound was a sea of unfamiliar faces as I was now a short timer. Steve's replacement arrived, Dr. Ron Witkowski. Ron had been in VN for five months, on a MILPHAP team near the Cambodian border. The 60-bed hospital didn't require three doctors and he was transferred to MACV. He was battle-tested.

Bob was shocked with Ron's nonchalant attitude as he described recoilless rifle attacks.

Bob wet his feet in Pediatrics, but the experience was more like swimming: three hours in clinic, followed by ward rounds. At lunch he shook his head, exclaiming, "The place is amazing.... I won't be able to change it. It'll change me! I ordered an IV for a kid to run 24 hours. I came back and it was done in two hours. It's like a big intensive care unit, but without nursing care. Parents provide the care. We had two kids die on the ward and another in the clinic. It's crazy!"

Pezzi leaned over the table to cheer him up, "Yes, Bob, in the delta where VC rule, it is like that *Life* magazine doctor Owen said, 'They die like flies and bleed like hell.'" Without a pause, Pezzi began speaking Italian. Bob is a proud Italian American and studied medicine in Italy. He immediately responded and the two enjoyed a long, animated conversation. The trick helped, just as it had with Woodruff speaking French to Vinh. After the Italian interlude, Bob's mood was sunnier.

Evening call was consumed by a 16-year-old girl who had been shot by a drunken soldier. Bob accompanied me to the ER, and we examined the girl. The bullet traversed her right lung. We inserted a chest tube, which helped her breathing, but the bottle rapidly filled with blood due to ongoing internal bleeding. A second tube led to the same result. We had no provision to open the chest to stop the bleeding. Her mother and sister held her hand with the IV. There was no power; a kerosene lamp and a candle lit the scene. Each time the girl breathed, more blood bubbled into the bottles. The mother squatted beside her, wiping her brow with a dirty towel. In the pale light, fear filled the mother's face. Bob and I followed the girl all night, but she expired at 5:00 a.m. The mother asked if the girl could remain in the ER until they arranged transportation. We covered her with an old blanket, and everyone tried to

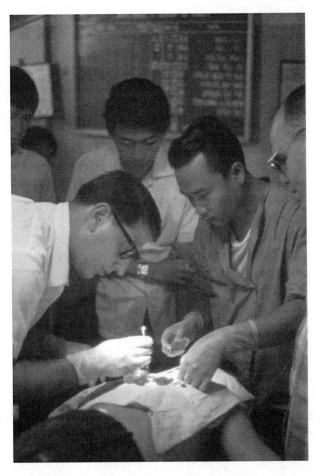

Dr. Bob Brittis operating on wounded VC, with VN nurses and Jim Jones on right.

sleep. In the morning the carpenter's hammer pounded shut the simple wooden coffin. The departed cargo was put on a cart that the family pulled from the hospital.

Vinh read a letter from the district chief of Gia Rai requesting an investigation of the deaths of six children. I told him we'd leave the next day.

We had a protective caravan for our risky drive to Gia Rai, complete with air escort, radio communication, and shotgun helicopter. As we entered the hamlet, we heard three explosions as ARVN engineers destroyed a canal block. Several loud bomb blasts followed the original explosions. Unfortunately, each time the block was destroyed, the VC conscripted civilian labor to rebuild, and airstrikes killed innocent workers.

Our investigation of the children's deaths revealed no mystery disorders. The fatalities were due to diarrhea, possibly cholera. We immunized a few dozen curious residents.

Hot weather persisted and the hospital was jammed with patients, especially children with diarrhea. Gia Rai had no corner on the market of the malady.

At 6:00 a.m. we heard distant explosions followed by the whoosh of F-100 jets attacking the canal blocks. Destruction from the air was tricky. In addition to civilian casualties, a bomb could damage the canal bank, flooding paddies and rendering the canal useless. It was a dilemma for General Minh. He employed antipersonnel weapons to harass the VC, who quickly retook the area as the ARVNs retreated. To

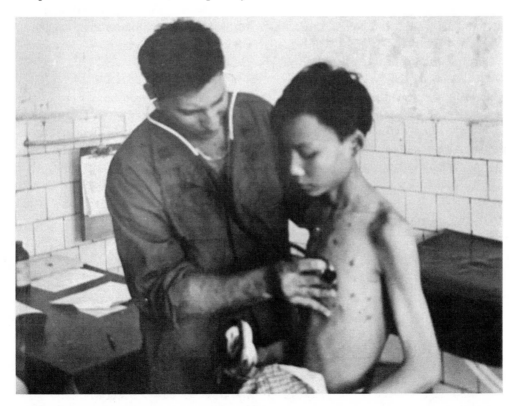

Dr. Bob Brittis examining boy with pneumonia who was cupped over his chest (photograph R. Brittis, MD).

permanently occupy the region would require many troops. The VC and the general were playing a lethal game of cat and mouse, but the VC had time and readily sacrificed civilians.

Jim returned from a week of R&R in Japan with a visible glow and tales of Tokyo's bustle. I received my orders and would depart to the United States on October 26. I was anxious to return and pick up my life. To be cool, well fed, clean, and unafraid would be a welcome relief.

My thoughts were bittersweet. I regretted my oft clumsy medical efforts, and our meager progress. Walking through the hospital, it seemed we had marched time for a year. We administered medicine to the suffering and tended their wounds, but had we achieved anything that would endure? I knew that despite our primitive facilities, I saved more lives than I would for years in the States. But what could have been accomplished with better equipment, additional personnel—a real hospital? And the war crippled our efforts. Public health was a disaster that we could not alter despite the work of dedicated USAID staff. Would there be any legacy? I consoled myself: regardless of the frustrations and challenges, I would gladly return. Our team achieved many medical successes and my relationship with Dr. Vinh was a marvel. I remained in awe of his stamina and dedication; he was key to the hospital's future. I wondered if Vinh's emphasis on cement buildings and roads represented permanence, as the war and Saigon's inefficiency eroded most of his plans.

Historians have given MILPHAP and other civilian medical programs mixed reviews. As the war intensified, MILPHAP teams increasingly focused on surgery as civilian casualties mounted. Fighting also affected the AMA Volunteer Physicians program, which was curtailed, and ultimately terminated, because of risk to AMA doctors. An impressive team of physician-administrators led USAID's efforts. Colonel Moncrief oversaw the civilian health program and was senior advisor to the MOH. He was ably supported by Drs. Douglas and Marsh, two talented and dedicated physicians who battled MOH's inefficiency and corruption. They ensured a constant supply of physicians and the four USAID nurses. But massive funding and talented administrators could not achieve USAID's goals.

The physician-historian Dr. Robert Wilensky wrote:

> The question to be answered is whether having all of these physicians running around the countryside to care for the indigenous population was worthwhile in terms of both the medical care provided and advancing the aims of the government of the United States.... It is difficult ... to quantify medical benefit to a civilian population during a conflict.... There were problems with supplies, in terms of both replacing and safeguarding them. Many hospital supplies appeared on the black market, and many were discovered with captured enemy soldiers.... there were [also] difficulties with VN physicians accepting the presence of the teams.... Providing direct care results in only temporary relief of the medical situation and contributes little or nothing to long term improvement in the health system.

But Wilensky acknowledged: "The MILPHAP program delivered quality medical care, and many Vietnamese civilians derived great and life-long dividends from it.... The success of the MILPHAP concept was attested to by the fact that other free world nations deployed similar teams to Vietnam, both military and civilian."

General Neel arrived at similar conclusions: "Despite the valiant efforts of the

U.S. teams, augmented by those from New Zealand, South Korea, the Philippines, and other nations of the free world, the broad and ambitious aims of PHAP could not be realized. The task of substantially improving health care in an under-developed nation was difficult enough. Compounded by civil strife and guerilla warfare, it became impossible."

It was a challenging year. I had treated bizarre diseases and battle wounds with antiquated medical facilities and bore witness to the Vietnamese citizen who suffered unspeakable hardships with resolute humility. The struggle against malnutrition, infections, poor education, and lack of preventive medicine was magnified by the government's inefficiency, corruption, and especially the war. Civilians were torn between supporting a political system that did not value their welfare versus the utopian promises of the VC, which were belied by their ruthlessness. Individuals such as Vinh were rare and vastly outnumbered by corrupt bureaucrats.

Any success had come at a price. The waste of lives and resources was staggering. I entered my last month in Bac Lieu with a mixture of sadness and relief.

Chapter Sources

Robert J. Wilensky. "The Medical Civic Action Program in Vietnam: Success or Failure?" *Military Medicine* 166, no. 9 (2001): 815–9.

_____. *Military Medicine to Win Hearts and Minds: Aid to Civilians in the Vietnam War.* Lubbock, TX: Texas Tech University Press, 2004.

Office of International Health. *Report on the Health, Population and Nutrition Activities of the Agency for International Development, 1966/1967.* U.S. Department of Health & Human Services Public Health Service, 1967.

Spurgeon Neel. "Corps Services." Chapter 12 in *Medical Support of the U.S. Army in Vietnam 1965–1970.* Washington, D.C.: U.S. Government Printing Office, 1973.

15

October

Midnight Madness, Medals, and Adieu

Morning clinics were busy, although the hospital would close for Confucius' birthday. On the holiday's eve, vendors hawked banana ice cream and sandwiches outside the building. The evening was Bob's first call and he had been to the hospital several times by dinner, when he exclaimed, "Jeez, this is worse than clinic. I've seen 20 kids so far and they keep coming." He continued excitedly, "One woman brought a baby this afternoon—the kid was stone cold. It'd been dead for hours. When I told her, the mother grabbed the kid, yelling and screaming, blaming me. I don't understand these people." Bob was struggling with the initial frustration and depression we all had experienced.

Following the holiday, the division conducted an operation near Gia Rai. Dr. Toch accompanied ARVN forces for a taste of battlefield action. The action was light but marred by an accident. An APC drove into a canal, tipping over and drowning two ARVN soldiers.

Jim spent the evening resuscitating a woman after a cardiac arrest. The midwives began mouth to mouth breathing and chest compression, which initially led to return of blood pressure and pulse. The woman had eight children, and soon a large family assembled as CPR continued. Jim intubated the patient and established a primitive breathing device, but blood pressure was unstable and the patient remained unresponsive. The family knew it was hopeless and asked to take her home. Jim removed the tube from her airway and the family carried the body to a waiting cyclo. The scene had been repeated hundreds of times over the past few months.

As excitement in maternity ebbed, more trauma arrived. A bus brought a girl of eight to the ER. She was walking near an outpost with her father, a PF soldier. Her father tripped a grenade used as a perimeter defense, with devastating results. These were primitive devices—hand grenades tied on wires or strings and strung around an outpost. The father was killed outright, and the girl sustained multiple wounds. Vinh and Pezzi worked for several hours and two PF soldiers donated blood. Despite these heroic efforts, she died.

After completing my nightly typing, Charlie, Bob, and I were enjoying a drink in the officers' club when two men entered and walked to the bar in the next room. A few minutes later we heard loud voices. Bob investigated and returned, exclaiming,

"You should listen to those guys—they're crazy!" He continued, "One is a USAID guy, the other is MACV. They're both drunk but want to drive to Ca Mau tonight."

Charlie opened the door a crack and we listened. The USAID official was complaining about lack of security: "Hell, this damn place is not pacified and we're too chicken to stick our heads out to show the VC we're not afraid of them." The officer agreed with his colleague but kept falling asleep and sliding off the barstool. The partner was warming to his point, "So why don't we show 'em tonight—let's really do it, old buddy. Let's show these candy asses it's as safe as driving downtown in the States."

Before the officer could respond, Bob burst into the room, yelling, "No, you guys can't do that—you are both drunk and it isn't safe."

"How long have you been in country?" asked the officer who was now awake and sitting upright.

"Long enough to know it isn't safe." responded Bob.

"Well, the hell with you, I've been here seven months."

The argument continued for a few minutes but ended abruptly as the duo stalked out of the club. We thought they were returning to their quarters, but they walked to the motor pool where they commandeered a jeep and the officer fetched two submachine guns from his hooch. Bob heard the commotion and trotted to the motor pool to stop them, but they drove past him to the gate where the bewildered guard attempted to dissuade them. They pushed him aside, opened the gate, and drove into the night.

Charlie alerted the duty officer, who awakened the commander. At this point it was not certain if the men intended to merely drive to the airport and back or planned to motor across the delta to Ca Mau, a dangerous journey of many miles. A major called a shotgun pilot to fly over the road in search of the wayward pair. The episode was now serious and potentially life-threatening.

Within a half-hour the pilot radioed the men were indeed proceeding toward Gia Rai, approximately 30 km distant, the first stop to Ca Mau. It was a dangerous situation: the road could be mined, or the VC would attack the vehicle. A detachment of the 1st Cavalry was encamped at Gia Rai and the commanding officer was called to set up a roadblock. We later learned the two avoided the roadblock, but drove their jeep into the canal, upon which the wet, drunken pair were arrested.

The following morning two hung-over individuals were called to face an angry colonel and their punishment. The episode was funny but tragic. They were lucky to survive their midnight escapade.

The weather turned rainy and cooler as Dr. Pezzi assumed weekend call, patching broken heads, and treating pneumonias and diarrheas, plus watching a young girl with typhoid fever slowly die of sepsis.

The colonel dictated new hooch assignments for no obvious reason. Officers carried tape recorders and bundles of personal items as they passed one another on the walkways. Hooch girls ferried other goods. Rain soaked those involved in the unnecessary exercise, another scene from Dowling's narrative.

The old Ba from Pediatrics died. She was a hospital fixture for nearly 20 years and beloved by the staff. A tearful Co Anh told me the Ba would herd relatives and animals out of the corridors, sweep the nurses' station, and clean the children's straw mats as she prepared food. A few days ago, Bac Si Tot saw her in clinic and admitted her. Jim subsequently examined her and diagnosed tetanus. The hospital had expended its supply of antisera, and the family were forced to buy the medicine from a local pharmacy at a huge price. But she received the drug late in the course of her disease. The slightest stimulus provoked tetanic seizures and coughing. She was awake and lucid to the end.

The following evening Charlie returned to the club after an ER call, cursing under his breath, "God damn suicide attempts—this one took 10 vitamin pills and was gorked!"

Bob asked, "What did you do, pump her stomach?"

"No, I gave her a shot and put her to bed. Her boyfriend showed up, so I left."

A couple of days later Vinh and I took a chopper to Gia Rai to meet Major Quyet, a combination provincial health worker and ARVN medical aid. A native of Hanoi, Quyet moved to South Vietnam in the late 1950s. Typical of many from the north, he was an energetic, highly charged individual who relished work. He made several suggestions to improve the hamlet's dispensary. Quyet's manner greatly pleased Vinh, who said the clinic was in good hands with him in charge.

Early the next morning, alarm clocks and telephones rang angrily, followed by a flurry of hooch activity. By 6:00 a.m. more than two dozen choppers were overhead, bearing the first wave of troops and advisors to Ca Mau. But there was little ground combat, and officers returned early. The day's tally was 30 VC casualties, plus 10 prisoners shot as the VC fled. By six o'clock MACV officers had showered, eaten dinner, and were at the bar or watching the evening movie. The episode reminded me of day camp.

Pezzi searched for a blood donor for an eight-year-old with GI bleeding. Several ARVNs volunteered to donate blood for 3,000 p. An angry Pio threw them out of the ER.

I flew to Can Tho to discuss the nursing shortage. USAID nurses were departing, and many VN nurses had been transferred to other facilities. We expected a group of student nurses, but the wards would be understaffed. Unhappily, USAID officials said we should not anticipate replacements.

Despite staffing problems, the hospital was busy. September statistics revealed 3,700 clinic visits, 55 major surgeries, 44 new cases of tuberculosis, and 70 war casualties, predominantly women or children—more than two war wounds a day. I recalled the slow pace of injured last November.

The fate of the "midnight wanderers" wasn't known, but we suspected the USAID worker would be transferred and the officer would receive disciplinary action, likely a fine and possible demotion.

More travel: I returned to Can Tho to give USAID representatives a recap of our year's activities and plans for my departure. Dr. Douglas handed me a copy of the latest USAID press release (Thursday, September 21, 1967): "Medical Team Reports on VN Health Programs." The article summarized the AMA's findings to President Johnson. The dedication of American health personnel was acknowledged, but the document highlighted the war, which hampered efforts to raise the quality of medical care, as well as the inefficacy of the Saigon government. The AMA concluded the number of hospital beds (18,000) was adequate but substandard, filled with infectious diseases due to lack of public health programs. TB, malaria, typhoid, dengue, cholera, plague, parasites, and other diseases ravaged the populace, especially children. Most water was contaminated, compounding the problems of sewage, lack of immunization, or control of rodents and mosquitoes. Public health education was essentially nonexistent, and doctors were limited by the war and the halting supply of medicines and equipment. Many doctors believed their government was more concerned with curative than preventive medicine.

It was a depressing report. I shook my head as Doug acknowledged its accuracy, wryly adding, "We've certainly got a lot of work to do." I agreed but wondered how much could be accomplished. The challenges were overwhelming.

After the meeting, MILPHAP representatives were treated to a Chinese dinner at the Red Cock restaurant. As we entered, our host said, "Boys, this is one of the few places in Can Tho where you can eat on the first floor, dance on the second, and on the third—well, we'd better eat first." The food was good, but little else.

In the morning, I returned to Bac Lieu with a boy I had seen in clinic a few weeks earlier. He was shot in the shoulder and referred to Can Tho for orthopedic surgery. Waiting on a bench with his mother, he squirmed and winced in pain. Luckily, the flight was not crowded, and the obliging USAID pilot let them board. When we arrived, I took them to the hospital and wrote a script for pain pills.

In my absence, Lt. Tom Johnson, MSC, replaced Don Robinson as our MSC administrative officer. Tom was a tall, blond lad from Mississippi with a pronounced southern drawl, and proud of it. He and Bob Brittis soon bonded. Tom had training in medical supply and logistics, an important asset to the team. His accent instantly betrayed his origins as he remarked, "I come from Texas, but I call Mississippi home, y'all."

A local hamlet chief and his son were assassinated. The province chief, General Minh, and the MACV commander met to discuss options. Two of the guilty were apprehended and security was strengthened. During the long VN conflict, thousands of local and national officials were assassinated. Partially offsetting the loss, a 75 mm recoilless crew were ambushed as they were setting up their weapon near Bac Lieu. A fierce firefight ensued with several VC killed, although their comrades escaped with the weapon.

Bac Si's Pezzi and Toch threw a champagne party in the officers' club. They invited hospital staff as well as MACV senior officers. Bac Si Vinh arrived but avoided the colonel. When Bob entered, the commander approached him, asking, "Well Doc, now that you've been here a couple of weeks, what do you think of the province? Have you gotten out to see the country yet? That's where the real action is."

Brittis smiled and picked an olive from a dish on the table, "Oh yes, colonel, I went downtown last night."

"No, no, I meant into the country—on a MEDCAP," emphasized the colonel.

Bob looked at him, responding, "Sorry Sir, but I've been too busy in the hospital." He nodded politely and walked away as the senior officer shrugged his shoulders and began another conversation. As many commanders, he believed MEDCAP

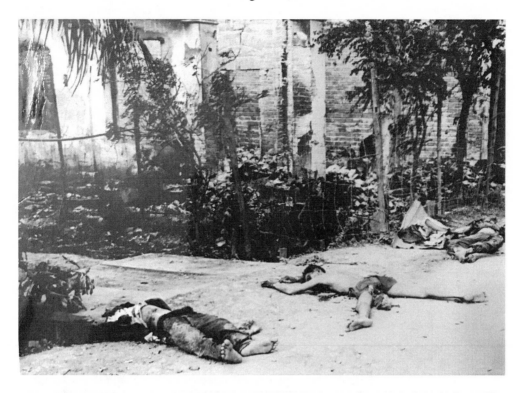

Ambushed VC casualties (unidentified VN photographer, sent to author).

programs were crucial, although their medical benefit was negligible. But one benefit of these "one-shot" hamlet visits was literally "shots"—immunization. Bob was beginning to understand the military mind.

Charlie and Jim had shared the same hooch for longer than Charlie lived with his wife before VN. They joked about ordering a double mosquito net and moving their bunks together. As we laughed, a Captain entered the club and announced the VC were shelling Phuoc Long. A new model of Spooky, "Super Spooky," was defending the town. The dragon ship carried the usual triple 7.26 mm gatling guns, but the latest version also had 20 mm cannons, which could deliver thousands of rounds in minutes. What a horrendous weapon. Charlie predicted morning would furnish the ER vivid results of "Super."

Dr. Vinh held a party for Pezzi and Toch, who would depart in a few days. After dinner the province chief showed slides from his recent trip to America. It was bizarre to watch tourist views of American cities, sitting in a Vietnamese home, awaiting an artillery barrage.

As I held clinic with Co Phuong, Dr. Vinh walked through the Dutch doors and exclaimed, "Bac Si Carlson. I have a surprise. You remember a few months ago you asked about cobra snakes?" I nodded in agreement, as I handed a script to Co Phuong. "Accompany me now," he exclaimed. "I have snakes today from Gia Rai. Come, I show you."

I protested mildly but Co Phuong said she would find someone to finish my clinic. Vinh drove me to his downtown office and we walked to the rear of the building. On the cement floor beside two frightened chickens were three black snakes, each at least four feet long. These "rang ho dat," or black cobras, were held by wire through their lower jaws. They squirmed as they fanned their hoods.

Vinh remarked excitedly, "You see, I get for you. Tonight, we have 'Chao rang ho'—cobra soup. Very good! You come at seven o'clock—OK?" I took pictures but avoided the writhing creatures on the cement as I nodded yes to his invitation.

That evening the MILPHAP physicians plus Pezzi and Toch drove to Vinh's house where a beaming medicine chief escorted us upstairs. He sensed our apprehension and plied us with cognac and wine. Vinh informed the group there are three varieties of cobra in Vietnam—"rang ho dat," the black cobra, or cobra of the earth; "rang ho hua," the night cobra, which is rumored to follow a lighted torch; and "rang ho may," the forest cobra, which can exceed 10 feet in length.

In a few minutes we were summoned to a circular table set with inlayed chopsticks, china soup bowls and spoons, together with embroidered linen napkins. Mrs. Vinh brought out a large tureen of a thick, green soup that smelled of lentils. A dish of boiled snake meat mixed with onions, garlic, and a spicy sauce was placed next to the soup. We were invited to sit. Mrs. Vinh served each a hefty portion of soup and the meat, plus soy sauce and vegetables. We initially hesitated, but were soon enjoying the food, which was very tasty.

After dinner Mrs. Vinh entertained us with her singing. As I listened, I saw a small lizard scurry across the wall chasing insects, I knew I would miss Vietnam, and especially the Vinhs. The exotic meal and music exemplified their hospitality and friendship during my year's sojourn.

Vinh drove Pezzi, Toch, and me to the airport and waved from the side of the strip as our Beechcraft traversed the runway, throwing mud and dirt in its wake. Vinh did not always bid farewell to volunteer physicians at the airport, but Pezzi and Toch, like Woodruff, Owen, and others, had made lasting impressions on the medicine chief. We flew to Saigon, where I made plans for Vinh's visit to San Francisco as Pezzi and Toch departed for America.

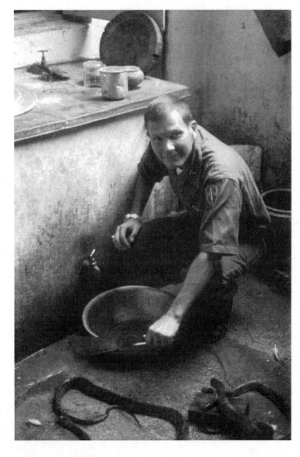

Cobras for dinner party and author at Vinh's office.

Rudolf Toch was born in Vienna. As a teenager he was imprisoned by the Nazis in the Dachau concentration camp for political offenses. He was freed in 1939 on condition he leave Germany, immigrating to New York and then to Massachusetts, where he graduated from Rollins College and Brown University School of Medicine. He became a U.S. citizen in 1944, served in the army in Korea, and was a pediatric oncologist at Harvard and Tufts medical schools. Toch published extensively and was an authority on childhood cancer. In describing his experience with kids in VN, he said, "There's nothing like the look in a child's eyes when he sees a balloon—in that respect the children there are just like American children." He was survived by a wife and two stepchildren (Rudolf Toch, MD, 1919–1999).

Pio Pezzi's father was a famous air force general who set altitude records. Pio graduated from a Rome medical school in 1953, followed by a Fulbright scholarship to the United States, where he completed surgical residency. He was a towering figure for many years at Abington Hospital, Pennsylvania. He married another physician and inspired generations of surgeons he taught. Pezzi had four children, including three physician sons. A few months before his death he recorded this message to a son: "I was reading my letters from Vietnam … it transports me so vividly to that place … it was a cesspool, but I was glad to have been there. You know, I helped some people, and I think I helped myself too … it gave me a view, a real view, of life" (Pio Pezzi, MD, 1927–2015).

I spent two days arranging logistics for Vinh's trip. When I returned to Bac Lieu, Tom Johnson drove me to the hospital gate where I saw the stakes and cement forms for the new driveway. Swarms of workers picked their way over piles of sand, rock, and cement. An excited Vinh acted like a straw boss. He saw me and extended a hand, "A present for you before you leave—the town provided money to finish the road. It will be completed before you depart. Isn't it wonderful?"

A new volunteer physician arrived while I was in Saigon: Dr. Tom Barrett, a generalist from Southern Illinois. A middle-aged fellow with a large pipe clenched between his teeth and a small doctor's bag, he was busy in surgery when I met him.

Friday the 13th proved to be unlucky for Bob, who was kept awake with a dozen hospital calls. Four children died and several critically ill patients were admitted. Bob took the losses badly.

Construction of the hospital road was now nearly complete. Most of the wooden forms had been filled with cement.

My night call was equally busy. At 11:00 p.m., I was summoned for a child with a bowel obstruction. We placed a nasogastric tube, which yielded an eight-inch ascaris worm, but the young girl died within an hour. A few minutes passed and I glanced at the body, which remained on the ER table. Three worms crawled from the nose of the dead child. The mother was standing beside the girl but didn't appear particularly concerned by the grisly sight. I admitted several other patients, with four deaths, including the girl with worms.

The following night was a pleasant contrast. The chief of police hosted a farewell dinner for me. The party included Vinh, two VN colonels, the province chief, and several local dignitaries, including the owner of the whore house, who greeted me warmly. My hosts were gracious and the meal delicious.

I spent the next morning writing reports and evaluations. The workers had completed the road project and covered the wet cement with tarps as it began to rain. Jim received an unexpected accolade from the MOH for the family planning clinic, an honor he greatly appreciated. Apparently, the efforts of the chief midwife and Dr. Lui had been successful—the clinic had not only been approved, but lauded. A party was held in maternity to celebrate. Champagne flowed and the midwives giggled after their second glass. The maternity clinic that followed was a happy affair. Jim tried to maintain his composure but couldn't help showing his happiness.

Unfortunately, the loop clinic did not survive. Jim was abruptly transferred to another MACV location shortly after my departure and Charlie completed his VN obligation soon thereafter. Bob was not involved in the maternity service. Hence, there was no ongoing source of IUDs or physician supervision. Years later, Bob told me the clinic simply closed. It was a noble experiment but may have been a precursor of the future. Birth control is currently widely available in Vietnam and the IUD one of the most popular methods of contraception.

Co Anh left for a second trip to Saigon. She would marry a pilot in November. She was terrified, but it was her only mechanism to secure a U.S. scholarship. Her mother would not give permission to travel unless she was married. Charlie gave his best premarital advice, but she was afraid of sex. When a VN couple became engaged, custom permitted a trial of intimacy before marriage. During her first trip to Saigon, she was introduced to her life's partner and participated in marital relations, which she disliked. Charlie reassured her she would learn to enjoy lovemaking and counseled her gently. The second time she returned from Saigon, she had a smile on her face, and a look of inner contentment, but told Charlie she was three weeks late for her period.

It rained throughout the day and mist obscured portions of the hospital. The EMs held a party for me, but I was on call and unable to trade shots of tequila with Sgts. Ray Vasquez and Jim Parker. Nevertheless, we recounted many Bac Lieu adventures, and I looked forward to our reunion in Texas. At eight o'clock, I examined an elderly man with acute appendicitis and called Vinh. The Bac Si arrived, and we stood under the cement fascia of the building avoiding the rain. We watched cows graze between the buildings. The scene seemed natural and peaceful. The patient squatted beside us on the cement as he held his abdomen, unafraid and resigned to the procedure. I tried to imagine my feelings eleven months earlier.

Two children I had admitted that day died, and another child with pneumonia was carried into the ER with a temperature of 105 degrees, heavily "cupped" and wrapped in three blankets plus a sweater. Previously, I would have been angry, but I removed the blankets and asked the family to buy some ice as I ordered antibiotics.

There was an ARVN operation, but no VC contact was made. I packed items to ship to the States and wrote MILPHAP reports. A ceremony was scheduled the next day to dedicate the new hospital driveway and I was to give a short speech.

The following morning, I finished my comments for the dedication and gave them to Co Phung to translate. At 9:00 a.m., the colonel summoned me to his office and presented me with the Bronze Star for meritorious service.

A few minutes later I was in front of the hospital to speak to the assembled crowd. I thanked those who contributed to the road and all who aided our efforts throughout the year. Co Phung repeated my words in Vietnamese. Polite applause followed. The province chief walked to the podium and bid me to stay at his side. His comments were brief and he turned to me. I was shocked as he shook my hand and pinned the First-Class Vietnamese Honor Medal on my breast pocket. The clasp was faulty, and the pin briefly pricked my chest as he attached the medal. Luckily, I only winced and made no sound as the assembled group applauded. His remarks ended the program. Several young girls in lovely *áo dàis* distributed refreshments. I was proud but stunned. Vinh came forward and patted me on the back as he grabbed my hand, followed by members of the city council, Jim, Charlie, and our EMs. Despite the early hour, cognac, beer, and whiskey were consumed at a brisk clip. Two hospital workers began clapping and dancing until Vinh gave a disapproving glance, which quelled their excitement.

We were restricted to the compound with a curfew, as local elections were scheduled the following day. During the September national elections more than 150 incidents were documented with considerable loss of life. Vinh scheduled a goodbye party for me the next evening.

My day was consumed with last minute packing and mailing. Dr. Douglas flew from Can Tho to wish me thanks and bid bon voyage. Although a curfew was in effect, the colonel gave us permission to attend Vinh's dinner.

Vinh's party was bustling by 6:00 p.m. The police chief, province chief, judge,

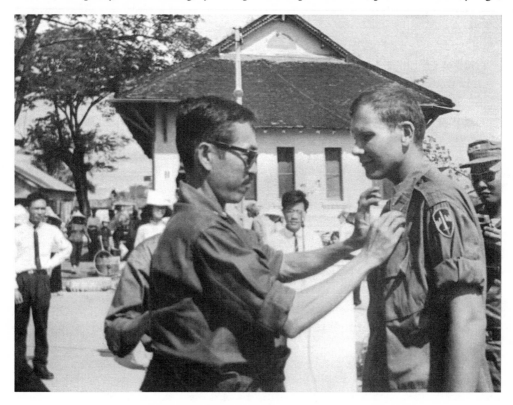

Vietnam Honor Medal Ceremony: province chief and author.

Dr. Douglas, Bac Si Tot and husband, our interpreters, and several hospital staff were socializing and sipping wine and cognac. Mrs. Vinh met me at the door in a lovely pastel blue *áo dài*. Vinh was serving drinks and mingling with guests. He gave me a one-armed hug and handed me a cognac. Dinner was a lavish affair: French onion soup, green salad, sweet-sour duck, creamed spinach and toast, fillet of sea bass, and dessert of butter cake with chocolate sauce. Each course was washed down with French wine, followed by cognac. After dessert, champagne was opened and we toasted everything—the country, the Vinhs, Dr. Douglas, and me. The evening ended with ginger tea. I bid farewell to the hospital staff, Mrs. Vinh, and Dr. Douglas, who thanked me for my service. It was short ride to the compound.

The evening ended with a final hooch dialogue. For 10 months Jim was friend, teacher, and mentor. Our evening chats had been wide-ranging, exploring literature, philosophy, medicine, and clinical research. He was a convincing spokesman for science, an accomplished investigator and excellent clinician. I benefited from his insight and knowledge. He asked of my plans. I told him I would enter a PhD program in physiology and pursue a career of clinical research, academics, and care of the needy. He was elated and we discussed my options. Rain pelted the hooch as howitzers provided the thunder for an otherwise gentle storm. I gave him a farewell embrace and thanked him for his guidance. He was a remarkable physician and friend. The two individuals who dominated my VN odyssey were Jim and Dr. Vinh.

The evening's howitzer bombardment was more than routine, as the guns were responding to attacks on local outposts. As I walked to the hospital the following morning, soldiers were unloading several coffins onto carts for the trip to the morgue on the new cement driveway. Nearly a dozen soldiers had been killed. The war hadn't paused for my benefit.

It didn't feel like my last day. I went through the motions of saying goodbye as I distributed gifts to nurses and hospital staff. It was difficult to believe I'd never see them again or know their fate. I bid farewell to Jim and Charlie, who wished me bon voyage, and gave Bob my best wishes as the team's new MOC. He was adapting and would be an effective leader of the team. I signed out of post and paid my hooch girl her monthly stipend plus a healthy tip. Tom Johnson loaded my baggage into a jeep, and we drove to the airport. Joan, Co Phung, MILPHAP corpsmen, and Dr. Vinh were waiting on the tarmac.

We chatted and reminisced until the 440 'bou circled the field and landed. The big, ugly plane taxied to the end of the field and opened its tail. EMs unloaded mail and cargo. Several VN strained at a rope retainer, waiting to board. The crew chief barked a curse at them, and they retreated slightly, but maintained their eagerness. I had priority as a PCS returnee. Tom and our EMs tossed my gear in the plane and saluted me. Although routine, I was moved by the gesture.

Bac Si Vinh looked at me and our arms locked. He grasped me with both hands. We did not speak and there was nothing I could say. Jim Parker yelled from the plane to hurry if I wanted a good seat.

"I must go, Bac Si," I finally blurted as I tried to relax his grip. He nodded. I stammered, "There's no way to thank you Bac Si. The year has been good. You are a brave and kind man who has taught me much and treated me as a son. When you come to the States, we will meet. And when I return to Vietnam, we will travel to Dalat. I must go. Thank you, Bac Si, 'Cam on ban.'"

He was silent but kept shaking my hand until I was forced to turn and walk to the plane. The rear hatch closed, and we taxied down the muddy, short strip for the last time. My final glimpse of Bac Lieu's medicine chief was Vinh standing as usual, slightly stooped, hands in pockets, with an ever-present cigarette dangling from a corner of his mouth as his eyes focused on the aircraft.

Goodbye Bac Si Vinh ... Adieu Bac Lieu.

Chapter Sources

United States Agency for International Development. "Summary of Six Man AMA Appraisal Team to President Johnson." News Release. September 21, 1967.

Rudolf Koch. Obituary. *Boston Globe*, December 1, 1999.

Christopher Pezzi, MD. Pio Pezzi's last voice mail, May 2015. Personal communication to author. January 10, 2020.

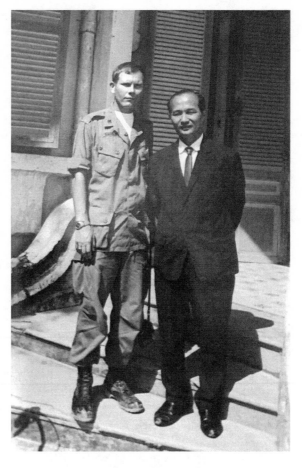

Author and Dr. Vinh.

Epilogue

Healing the Wounds

My return to the United States coincided with John McCain's capture in Hanoi by North Vietnamese, who downed his A-4E Skyhawk jet with a SAM missile on October 26, 1967. My military duty ended six months later; McCain would endure imprisonment and torture for five and a half years.

Following two weeks' leave I returned to Fort Sam Houston, where I taught corpsmen bound for Vietnam. For an interval I maintained frequent correspondence with the Bac Lieu team, but soon most of my colleagues rotated home. I learned the savagery of the 1968 Tet offensive horror from Bob Brittis, who wrote Bac Lieu was irreversibly altered by that event.

On discharge from active duty, I applied to graduate school as a PhD candidate in physiology. USC was fortunate to have two pioneering faculty—Dr. Max H. Weil, the "Father of Critical Care Medicine," and Dr. Findlay Russell, an early leader in toxinology, the study of venoms. I became a student under Dr. Russell's supervision. During medical school and OB residency, I had worked with Dr. Weil in the Shock Research Unit at LA County, where computers were first used to monitor patients. As I served in VN, Weil selected my fiancé Barbara Bailey as a head nurse for the new USC Center for the Critically Ill. Upon learning of my status as a graduate student, Weil generously offered me access to his research facility and participation in the lab's studies of ICU topics, a relationship that blossomed over the next decade.

I set my research goal on the study of marine venoms and the stonefish of Australia's Great Barrier Reef, one of the most dangerous animals in the world. However, my desire for a South Sea adventure was dashed, although a Naval accident became a lucky break. The famed undersea explorer and inventor of the aqua lung, Jacques Cousteau, developed a subsurface chamber where investigators could live and work for extended periods of time. It was the equivalent of an underwater "space station" and received extensive press coverage. The Navy had a similar underwater project, SEALAB, near San Clemente Island, California. Scott Carpenter, the astronaut hero of the Mercury Project, combined space and undersea exploration. Carpenter had worked with Cousteau and was a guiding force in the development of SEALAB. During one dive he was stung by a sculpin, a common fish that congregate near pilings and underwater structures. The sculpin's official name is the California scorpionfish, and its spines contain a venom like the deadly stonefish. Sculpin stings are not life-threatening, but intensely painful, and potentially lethal 50 feet beneath the surface. Carpenter survived the incident, but headlines proclaimed: "Astronaut Stung by Poisonous Fish." My mentor, Fin Russell, had contracts with the Office of Naval Research for the study of other marine venoms and utilized the incident for additional support. I became the lucky recipient and was awarded Navy funding and a fellowship. The research entailed collecting still-flopping fish from a dock in San Pedro from a wizened Italian fisherman, followed by a hurried trip to our lab to extract and stabilize the precious venom for studies. I was occasionally stung as we pipetted tiny drops of the poison from the spines, but a compensation was the ability to eat our tasty specimens. Naval funds provided tuition, equipment, and supplies, reducing my need to moonlight in LA's emergency rooms.

In late 1968, I visited AMA headquarters in Chicago to produce the film "Bac Si My," a recruiting tool for volunteer physicians.

Barbara and I were married in 1969 as men walked on the moon, a union that endured nearly 51 years. I was anxious to complete my PhD. In addition to venoms, we studied shock, respiratory failure, and other life-threatening disorders. I loved research, but the underserved remained a priority. Jim's comments of marrying research opportunities with clinical service proved correct. I remained at USC and LA County after my PhD for training in internal medicine and critical care, where I developed a third allegiance—teaching. The evolving field of critical care medicine allowed me to practice medicine, pursue clinical research, and teach physicians and nurses. Dr. Weil offered me a position as clinical director of the USC Center for the Critically Ill and a faculty appointment in the medical school.

The years sped by. It was exciting to be at the dawn of a new field of medicine, working with physicians, nurses, and others with a shared a vision of intensive care. My training in physiology was the perfect grounding for a career in critical care: to understand how disease or injury affects organ systems and to integrate comprehensive management. Memories of VN faded, although psychological wounds lingered. I didn't discuss Bac Lieu and it was painful to be reminded of the war. I avoided reading my journal.

In the late 1970s I moved to Detroit and Wayne State University, a professorship, and the opportunity to develop a multihospital critical care service and training program.

We published papers, chapters, and textbooks as I climbed the academic ladder and the burgeoning field of critical care medicine, culminating in my election as president of the Society of Critical Care, current professional home to more than 16,000 multidisciplinary intensive care practitioners. I later moved to a University of Illinois College medical campus as department chairman, followed by 25 years at Maricopa Medical Center (now Valleywise), the county hospital of Phoenix, professor at Mayo Clinic College of Medicine and the University of Arizona College of Medicine, and governor for the American College of Physicians. I have had a rich career and the joy of working with and teaching hundreds of physicians, nurses, and other health professionals.

My clinical activities slowed, and Barbara urged me to review my Vietnam journal and contact my Bac Lieu colleagues. The hunt has been hampered by the elapsed decades. As Vinh predicted, many have "passed to the west," and it has been impossible to write their epitaphs, but tracing the lives of the healers became a quest.

I met Dr. Vinh for the last time in late 1968. He was completing his surgical tutorial in San Francisco and asked if we could meet at Disneyland. A few days later we spent several hours at the California theme park. He was fascinated by the exhibits and bought souvenirs for his family, exclaiming, "It is like a real city, but make-believe." Late that afternoon we stood at the entrance gate, once again shaking hands as Mickey and Donald greeted visitors to the Magic Kingdom. I don't recall our final comments, and soon he was escorted by a USAID representative to a waiting car. I never saw him again.

Steve Reynard completed training and practiced cardiology in the coastal community of Dana Point. I interacted briefly with Steve in the 1980s when he recalled his family's vacation to Bac Lieu. He told me a few of the hospital staff remembered the tall Bac Si from California. Years later I spoke with Dr. Francis Reynard, Steve's widow, who recited Vinh's immigration to Southern California. Dr. Vinh visited Steve once or twice, but subsequent contact was lost. Steve had a successful medical practice, working with Fran, a pediatrician. They had three sons. Approximately a dozen years ago Steve developed Parkinson's disease, related to Agent Orange exposure—with a long and ultimately fatal course (John S. Reynard, MD, 1938–2019).

The hunt for Charlie Gueriera was facilitated by an alumni association, Drexel University, which superseded Hahnemann Medical College, Charlie's alma mater. After Vietnam, Charlie completed Ob-Gyn residency and practiced in Pennsylvania and Virginia. He was an avid hunter and fisherman and donated generously to free clinics and humanitarian causes. He had five sons (Charles Gueriera, MD, 1937–2005).

Joe Neal resumed medical school at Stanford, graduating in 1970, followed by general surgery and cardiothoracic training in New Mexico. He returned to Modesto, California, and an illustrious career in cardiovascular surgery, with marriage and two children. He retired recently. Joe had fond memories of Jim, Dr. Toch, Vinh, and the MILHAP team. He worked on the medical ward and participated in the management of patients with advanced TB. He related the tale of a venerable Chinese gentleman who stoically allowed the young student to perform a chest procedure. Joe was amazed at Jim's encyclopedic medical knowledge, surgical expertise, and love of teaching.

My attempts were unsuccessful to learn the future of the four USAID nurses, Don Robinson, and our corpsmen.

The fate of the elusive Dr. Jones was difficult to uncover. We scoured records at UC San Francisco and Berkeley, as I assumed Jim returned to the Bay Area after Vietnam, but our efforts yielded no results. Bob Brittis ultimately clarified the story. Jim was transferred from Bac Lieu to another setting in VN in late 1967. Bob lost touch with him, although he knew Jim was a fellow New Yorker. On discharge from the Army, Jim returned to New York, initially at Westchester Medical Center, where he contacted Bob. Jim resumed his academic career and made important contributions to reproductive medicine and infertility as professor of obstetrics at Downstate Medical School and the Robert Wood Johnson Medical School, and chairman emeritus at New York Medical College. He was married three times with several children and grandchildren. Jim died of a cardiac arrest at age 72 in Florida. His obituary was published in the *New York Times* (James R. Jones, MD, 1935–2007).

Bob Brittis survived the Tet offensive and successfully led the MILPHAP team throughout 1968. He practiced pediatrics for many years, raised a family, and is retired in New York.

As the Bac Lieu alumni pursued their lives, the war churned and escalated, adding more wounds to Vietnam's citizens. Following the bloody 1968 Tet offensive, the VC's strength was sapped and the North Vietnamese People's Army of Vietnam (PAVN) dominated the war. To end the conflict, Lyndon Johnson vowed not to run for reelection in 1968 and halted bombing of North Vietnam. However, the assassination of Robert Kennedy ended the most likely Democratic presidential campaign and drove a stake through the heart of the peace movement. Barbara and I supported Bobby Kennedy during the California primary and watched his acceptance speech on TV and the confused scene after he was shot. A surgeon friend rendered aid to the mortally wounded senator, who was carried from the Ambassador Hotel to Good Samaritan Hospital, a short distance from us. In their final moments, both JFK and RFK were cradled by physician acquaintances. Years later I knew Dr. Tom Shires, who tended John Kennedy's gruesome injuries in Dallas.

After Robert Kennedy's death, Hubert Humphrey could not compete with the law-and-order candidacy of Nixon, who was elected president in November 1968. Nixon's bid had been clandestinely aided by Anna Chennault, widow of the famed World War II Flying Tigers general. With Nixon's blessing, she secretly maneuvered the South Vietnamese delegation to stall the Vietnamese Paris peace accords, a final blow to Humphrey's chances. In the early 1970s, Nixon began unilateral withdrawal of American forces, leaving the South Vietnamese regime to bear the sole burden of the war. In June 1972, the nation's attention briefly shifted from Vietnam to the Watergate episode, culminating in impeachment hearings and Nixon's resignation in August 1974. America's withdrawal continued during that interval and was nearly complete by 1973, although fighting continued until April 1975, when Saigon fell to PAVN and Gerald Ford declared America's presence in Vietnam had ended. A frantic evacuation of civilians ensued, including the Vinh family. President Thieu resigned and excoriated America as he fled to Taiwan. Despite its strength and massive effort, the United States lost the war. The severity of American social unrest related to VN has been compared to the American Civil War.

The allegory of Vietnam's wounds continued and evolved. Vietnam treated its country's citizens harshly. During the latter stages of hostilities and beyond, civilians endured untold suffering. There is little record of the transition of provincial medical care, but many medicine chiefs probably fled the country as had Dr. Vinh, or were "retrained" to work under the communist regime. Thousands of physicians, nurses, and other health professionals faced a difficult choice. Disruption of provincial life was severe, but the upheaval was not documented. Nevertheless, the health of Vietnam's citizens has progressively improved, and its population has risen to more than 95 million. Current estimates of preventive medicine, nutrition, and other measures of public health are positive, although it is impossible to estimate the human cost to achieve those goals. Vietnam remains a communist country, with ongoing issues of human rights, but is an active trading partner with the United States and a popular destination for American tourists. We have a habit of befriending former enemies. Ho Chi Minh's dream of an independent communist Vietnam has been realized.

What of America's wounds? The war began with a fallacy—the domino theory of communist aggression. The conflict ended with lies and deception—some say betrayal. But the Saigon regime was corrupt and lacked the trust of its citizens, whereas the VC and the North were steadfast in their commitment. Debates will continue, but the war is over. The ultimate trauma to those who died can never be erased, and returning veterans were met by a confused America that blamed its soldiers for the sins of their leaders. Our nation was irreversibly scarred by the episode. Vietnam's legacy yet resonates, as the war heralded a loss of faith in government, exacerbated by subsequent events in Iraq and Afghanistan. These salted America's wounds, adding their own physical and psychological lesions to the U.S. psyche.

But injuries heal, albeit slowly. Decades have elapsed and two generations have learned of the conflict from books and movies. The most passionate have died or mellowed and the war is increasingly examined with the 20–20 hindsight of history. Hopefully, the United States will be more forthright in future military adventures. Trust must be earned, but I am cautiously optimistic.

My wounds have been salved by time and reviewing this memoir. For years, I transported the yellowed pages of my journal from house to house, relegating them to a corner of a garage. Time had dulled my aversion to the narrative, although I was amazed as I read passages written decades ago. Did I do and see those things? But for many sections, I could predict the next scene. People, places, and dialogues raced to my consciousness and I was transported a half-century earlier.

Reliving my year in Bac Lieu has been a healing and learning process. I recounted my colleagues' commitment to treat Vietnam's citizens, documenting our struggles in a single hospital for one year. But many Vietnamese as well as PHAP teams, AMA physicians, military doctors, nurses, corpsmen, and countless others gave solace. Despite the horror, confusion, and the war's conclusion, my odyssey reaffirms individuals will aid those in need despite overwhelming odds. And that is a reason for hope.

Chapter Sources

Charles J. Gueriera. Obituary. *Potomac News & Manassas Journal Messenger*, March 2, 2005.
James R. Jones. Obituary. *New York Times*, February 14, 2007.
John S. Reynard. Obituary. *Orange County Register*, February 23, 2020.

Index

211